Foreword

I was fortunate enough to be one of the first people to train with Bob Burns and his 'Swan'. I remember thinking at the time that this was a game changer. The ability to have informal chats with the subconscious mind made therapy not only more effective but also a lot more enjoyable to engage with.

Over the years I've gotten to know Bob really well and can appreciate the breadth of his creativity, his experience, his story telling and his easy-going affable style that helps create irresistible rapport with clients.

This book is like attending a workshop with Bob. A born raconteur, Bob will delight you with his stories, his musings and reflections and explain how the Swan, which literally 'came to him' one day, developed into a major therapeutic modality taught around the world many years later. You are about to embark on a fascinating journey. Enjoy, and I'm sure you will get as much pleasure from listening to Bob as I and countless others have done.

Felix Economakis
CPsychol (Counselling Psychologist and creator of: 'The 4Rs Therapy')

REAL OR
IMAGINED

Hypnotherapy by
BOB BURNS

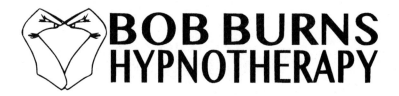

BOB BURNS HYPNOTHERAPY

First Published in 2021
Self Published by Bob Burns
Copyright © Bob Burns 2021
Written By Bob Burns
Cover design & Photography by Dean Rhymes
ISBN: 9798741581162

Video QR Codes

There will be a chance to view demonstration video clips, by using the QR codes displayed throughout this book. Simply scan the QR codes on the following pages, using a QR code scanner app on your mobile device, this will take you directly to the video content.

The web links are also available at the back of this book for those who would prefer to use them.

Contents

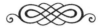

There were a little over 200 Gods sitting in the small amphitheatre. They were excited. Theus hadn't addressed them for some time and they had always enjoyed his wisdom. His ideas. His games. And so, a bolt of lightning struck the marble stage and suddenly there he stood, resplendent in a golden cape. Theus did have style and had always liked entrances. He smiled, "I have decided to send him... A Swan!" Acromites stepped forward, bowed slightly and asked, "But what will The Swan do?" Theus answered, "It will open a Gateway, but only for those who come to understand it."

CHAPTER 1

Hello Reader

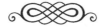

This is a book about clinical hypnotherapy. How you liking it up to now? I know it's early days but do you get a *sense* of who I am yet? Have we already met, or had you heard *of* me or perhaps attended one of my workshops or been mentored by me before you bought this book? You did *buy* the book, didn't you?!!! For if not... the curse of *Zarak* can be a frightening thing!!!

I have no idea who you are of course. But I guess you will be either a therapist or someone considering learning hypnosis. Or perhaps someone seeking 'just one more thing' and hoping you can find it here? You might do, I'm fully trained an' everything! I could make all forms of assumptions but what I think might be for the best is to assume that you know nothing.

Yep, I can hear some groaning going on already ☺ LOL (yeah there's gonna' be lots of smiley faces & LOL's. I'm a modern-day writer?) But if I can explain, in the hypnotic world the skills and knowledge are 'all over the place', just as are the *claims* of skills and knowledge. So, if I can assume that you know very little (hopefully without at any time insulting your intelligence) I won't leave anything out. Obviously, I'm talking about *my* style, *my* protocols, the *how* and *why* of my work and not the 'history of hypnosis', which you can read online or go do a hypnosis course. Sometimes they spend a couple days dragging you through all of that until your ears bleed! Then you forget it all. Then you go online again to be reminded of it all on a Thursday night when you've got nothing to do. Then you post historical arguments in forums. I do remember doing this workshop some years ago and it went really well. In fact, so well that the person who had booked me to run it mentioned that I had actually 'over delivered'? They went on to remind me that many of the people attending were indeed my competition and that I had revealed some *stuff* that might have been better held back? I laughed and informed my sponsor that it probably didn't really matter *how* good I was, *what* I showed them and *how* much I revealed, as in my experience, *"they never use it anyway!"* I remember him looking puzzled at me, before I told him that many of the things I teach seem so crazy that many people smile, write it down, put it to one side with the intention they'll get round to it, but never do. Or I get the other type, who, when I ask months later, *"And are you having success with that thing I showed you?"* would often give me the good news that they *loved it*,

BUT they had now made it *even better* by adding this or that to it, and I would go *"Wow!"* and smile my loveliest smile (I have a lovely smile). Or they might inform me that they felt that that particular thing wasn't for *them* and again I would smile and nod (I have a lovely nod). The good news is I get messages every day from many people whom I have been so lucky and indeed honoured to have helped over the years in using some of 'that stuff' and how it works well for them. And of course, they lovingly share *their* ideas and concepts with me which I *always* try out, no matter how crazy. And much of it I do indeed keep! So, a big shout out to all those students who became members of my peer group before going on to teach and inspire *me* (and still do) on a regular basis. I do hope however, that you might still pick something up from this wee *tome*. Remember, *'Teaching is not just about new information. It can also be about being reminded of something wonderful which you already knew, but forgot along the way?'* ☺

CHAPTER 2

ME!

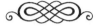

But let's do a very quick run down on me and my history, get that out of the way and then we can have some fun!

I left school at fifteen with The Scottish Leaving Certificate in English and Arithmetic (maths had not been discovered at that time). Served my time as a butcher. Had a shedload of labouring jobs from coalman to milkman to pick and shovel to demolition. But like I said I served my time as a butcher, owning my own shop for a few years and then got a sales job and started thinking about how people worked. Did a shedload of more sales jobs and got involved in financial services. Became consultant of the year then became Area, District and Regional manager of the year (over separate years obviously) before becoming National Sales Manager (looking back I was somehow always being over-promoted). I then studied psychology, sociology, the humanities and philosophy and got myself an honours degree in Social Science. Whilst doing all of the above I became a professional singer, magician and mentalist, eventually making a full-time living from these skills. I was also a cage dancer (rubber cage for safety in case of fire) in a nightclub in Barcelona where my nickname was 'El Leopardo' (The Leopard).

I should quickly say that one of the above is actually not completely true. I was also very heavily involved in what is best termed as Spiritual Healing and went on to train in a development circle, spending many years in darkened rooms holding hands with total strangers *(this was still linked to Spiritualism by the way)* I trained with The Samaritans, before realising that listening to someone's problems on 'the conscious level' was really not for me (no disrespect to The Samaritans who do a phenomenal job). I have worked with hypnosis on many levels and used it in stage shows, street, impromptu, during mentalism shows, during close-up magic and of course in the therapy room where I work as a full-time therapist. And that, in an extremely scattered nutshell, is the story of my professional life.

This book, as I said, is ostensibly about hypnosis and hypnotherapy. But hopefully there will be some interesting anecdotes, totally evidence based of course ☺ , and stories linked to other stuff along the way that will both make you think and hopefully smile. I love the idea that *'on little hinges swing big doors'* and I hope that I may be able to share some of these small stories that might have a bigger meaning for you in order to perhaps provide thoughts to steer by. The book's purpose will not be as a manual (*although there will be several protocols and thoughts within these pages that for me are truly golden*), but rather as a guide to my own particular model. I am experienced in many methods and models constructed by others and ALL of them are excellent but very few of them will be mentioned in this book. My findings are that the chances of getting a great result in the therapy room depends mainly on the *type* of therapist and where they are at that time of their therapeutic path. For me, assuming the proper training has taken place, experience plays a huge part, along with *activity knowledge* and *knowhow*, and of course talent will indeed play its part. I've always found it fascinating how therapists get to learn and experience different things at different times, very often totally unplanned. Grasping what suits them at one particular moment of their career whilst placing something on the shelf for use at a later date. Then when they look at it again, they wonder why they left it on the shelf in the first place. Maybe they simply weren't ready for it at that time? But in this book, I will mainly be leaning on my own model. The hypnosis and protocols that I *use* every day in my therapy room. And of course, the reasons *why* I use them. These are models I did not find in any book or written by someone who got their ideas by reading someone else's book based on another's model.

Painting the Perfect Picture

There is nothing wrong with using another's model. It's where we all have to start out. But for me it's a bit like painting a perfect picture. I mean it's easy enough to paint a picture isn't it? You can even paint a picture by numbers. You've seen those lovely books for children whereby if you want to paint a picture all you have to do is know that all the ones are red, all the twos are blue and all the threes are yellow. You stick the proper paint in the numbered spaces, try not to go over the lines and voila! You have a perfect picture which clearly reveals what it is. The only problem with it is that when you look at it you instantly know that none of it is *you*!

Rather you simply followed someone else's process. But if you really want to paint a picture that *is* you then you have to get lots of different paints, a paint brush and a palette with a blank canvas. Then you simply go and knock yourself out! You discover that if you mix the red and blue you immediately get purple, with red and yellow you have orange and blue with yellow creates green. And by adding more of one and less of the other then mixing in blacks and whites in order to create light and shade you find you can turn your palette into a virtual smorgasbord of colour including indigos, violets, tangerine, pink, brown, lavender, maroon and so forth and by applying them to your canvass you find yourself creating something that has never been painted before! Imagine that for a moment! Imagine creating something that has never been done before! Sure, it might not seem to be as perfect as when you were painting by numbers, but THIS painting is all...about...you! Your very own work of art! Having said that we might want to very quickly ask, 'what actually *is* a work of art'? Do you know? It's an interesting question... yes? Shouldn't we individually know the answer to that? I remember whilst studying philosophy at one point we touched on the *'philosophy of art'* where the professor asked a question which many philosophers will be aware of (philosophers love to read my work ☺). The question was this, *'Your 4 year old child has come back from nursery where they have painted something just for you! You look at it, you don't have a bloody clue what the hell it is and yet, you can feel your eyes burning and your chest swells with pride.*

Your baby's first offering! But now comes the question. (You may wish to think about this yourself. Be very brave okay?)... *"Can this creation from my 4-year-old child possibly be classed as a work of art'?"* And I can tell you that although many of the male students back then believed it was indeed *possible* nearly *all* of the females in that class felt that they somehow *knew* that the answer could only be a resounding YES! The professor smiled, then opened his mouth and gave the answer, which was quite interesting in itself because in philosophy, and social science in general, very often there are no actual *answers!* (I can just see the social scientists among you reading this and nodding their heads). I remember that many of these students of philosophy were totally and completely *pissed off* with his reply, He informed us that: "From the world of 'philosophy of art' we now believe that in order for a painting to be truly a work of art two things have to be considered. The first is, 'Was there a great skill involved in this piece?' And the second is that of 'intention'. Did this 4 year old child truly *intend* that this should be viewed as a work of art?"

So, over the top of the disagreement and indeed resentment met from the class (ain't philosophy fun?) The professor made it clear that a four year old probably would not have the skill, and even if they did it still could not *be* a work of art because the 4 year old child would have had no intention of it *being* so (hey guys, don't shoot the messenger! ☹). I actually loved this wee moment in my journey. I remember thinking that 'I will remember this forever' and up until now I have.

But back to where we are, developing the skills and having the intention to create our *own* works of art. Why not? I do indeed pick certain tools up now and again from the giants on whose shoulders I stand upon as it's a great idea to have several arrows in your quiver. But for me the best toolbox is always the one YOU build yourself. The best book is always the one YOU write yourself. And the best place to write that book is in YOUR therapy room. A place where you turn theory into fact. Or at least, strong *empirical evidence* that leads you closer to fact, assuming there is such a thing ☺ (the funny faces are annoying you by now yeah? Look, I'm running a social experiment here, get involved!). But I do believe all therapists share the same *raison d'etre* (yeah I speak Italian, so sue me!), that being to create a positive change in all of those who come to ask for our help. All else is surely narrative. You could even say we try to make a '*Change Phenomena*' (I do hope somebody writes that term down, possibly turning it into an event one day? Maybe I could be a guest speaker. As I said earlier, I'm fully trained and everything!).

What I DO

At this time of writing, apart from working as a clinical hypnotist most days in my therapy room, I deliver hypnotic workshops both here in the UK and all around the world.

It was suggested to me in writing this book that I might attempt to answer the very excellent question (I do believe from a certain Benjamin Pyatt)**, 'What makes you different?** I don't think a good instructor, teacher, writer, needs to be too different.

Skill is skill and flair is flair. But to the best of my knowledge I do believe there is something that I do that at this moment of writing I am not aware of anyone else who does this particular *thing*. I have also spoken to many skilled therapists from around the world and they also tell me that they know of no one else who does this or offers this particular service. Quite simply I teach therapy *in* the therapy room. That is, I mentor experienced therapists who get to come to work with me each day. I need to add very quickly that my clients are very happy to accept *visiting consultants*, who are here to see *me* and not the client. I should say however that if it is of a sexual nature or one that I consider to be of extreme anxiety I only work one-to-one with the client. So, the student comes with me into the therapy room. They are introduced to the client and that's it. They are not allowed to film or record, but they can take notes (only for our later discussion, then these notes will be destroyed). And of course, at the end of the therapy they are very welcome to ask any questions they wish. The clients seem to quite enjoy it actually, indeed it's almost like they are receiving even more attention? Two for one if you will. Which of course is true as now and again the visiting consultant may wish to contribute their thoughts at the end of the session. So, when someone contacts me for mentoring, I *don't* just sit down and talk hypnosis with them. I have no problem with any of my esteemed colleagues doing that but, for me, I insist that they come into my wee *pied-a-terre* of a therapy room and *see* what I do. That way they know that, a) I actually do what I say I do and exactly the way I say that I do it and b) It works.

Après Therapy

Later that evening, when we return from the therapy room I like to show my Highland Hospitality by cooking for my *mentee* and we dine and chat and sip health giving malt whisky and fine wine into the late evening, covering everything that happened that day and why. And of course, we look at some of the interesting cases that will come up the next day. Also, I will give them a private session or two if they so wish in order to work on any issues they might personally be carrying, and happily teach them all my main protocols during their visit. Later, when they have returned home and read all their notes and the material I give them, we have a Skype session where we get the chance to *wash up*. Here they also get the chance to ask about a case they possibly watched me work on the week previously and they will often be surprised on how that little thing we did got a complete result. I am very happy if they wish to follow up by talking to the client who, as I said, actually very often seem to enjoy the added attention, which I think is quite lovely.

[Actually in revisiting this chapter through Covid-19 having an effect on our work since February 2020 all my clients see me online which means my mentoring with clients in my therapy rooms have halted (meantime). Also workshops are now held online, which I am currently struggling with slightly because talking into a small camera with no 'volumed' reaction is soooooo draining! But as they say 'it is what it is'.]

If I may I would like to ask you the reader to be alert throughout this book and accept that in many of the stories within its pages I am NOT so much giving my views, beliefs, ideas, but rather I am merely reporting to you some of the truly amazing things which I have honestly witnessed in the therapy room and with people in general. Indeed, some of these stories will for some readers appear so totally absurd that, to be perfectly candid, I had a good long hard think with regard to whether or not I really wanted to share some of them. But they are here, in your hands. You can make of them whatever you will. But I do hope you, the reader, might find this book entertaining, as I reveal a little about me, where I came from, and of course why and how I do what I do.

You will also be aware that I was asked for some case studies to be included in this book… (case studies… *with insight as to how and why the therapist believes it worked*) … and I will indeed sprinkle a few throughout, which I hope will give food for thought, with regard to the amazing world of the human mind, which we as therapists get to view. So… let's have one right now shall we?

Case Study 1

George and The Dualler I mentioned earlier that the student in my therapy room gets to see how I work. They also get to see me appear to fail and what I do when that happens. This reminds me of the time when I had Anton, a visiting consultant from Belgium arrive at my home here in Montrose.

16

He very kindly informed me how excited he was to be able to see me work in the therapy room. The first case that morning was George, a local guy around 40 years old who had several anxiety issues, one of them being, "I get really anxious on The Dualler (his term for The Dual Carriageway) and just can't drive on it!" The problem being that the only way North or South of Montrose is The Dual Carriageway! I had already seen George for The Consultation the week prior, and hypnotically he came across as a poor subject. I never got even remotely close to hypnotising him or doing **The Swan** (we'll talk later about The Swan), Anyway I went through the notes with Anton prior to George's arrival for his second session. And when he arrived, I asked the opening question with regard to how he was and how things were since our last session. George of course informed me that there had been no difference to which I could see Anton slide down in his chair, probably thinking about the 1600 mile round trip to visit The Master (that's me by the way). And whether or not there might be a rebate? Anyway, I carried on regardless, eventually asking George what he had got up to over the weekend. He replied that he had gone to a show in Dundee. "Dundee?" I asked. "Can I ask how you got there?" And when George told me he had driven there I simply asked him, "And the return trip? Did you drive home?" And of course, George confirmed that he had done so. I then pretended to review his notes meticulously before gently informing him, "Y'know George, looking at your notes here I'm reminded that the main reason why you came to see me is because you can't drive on the dual carriageway, is that right?"

George stared at me before revealing, "Yeah...yeah... I drove to PERTH on Sunday!" I smiled, "That would be twice as far as Dundee, yeah?" "Yeah!" he answered, "Do you think you're fixed?" I asked. George thought long and hard, ".....I must be!" he replied, still staring through me. Anton was of course thrilled. It would appear I had become The Master once again. But let's have a look at this case. We have someone I cannot hypnotise and yet gets fixed very quickly. How is that possible? And the answer is that sometimes it's like that. The person does not have an ahaa moment. They don't scream "Eureka!" They don't punch the air because nothing has actually happened (consciously)! By that I mean that in many cases they simply become normal. And in becoming normal there is nothing to write home about. Indeed, they don't even recognise that they have *become* normal. Quite simply, the skilled therapist said something and she said it in a certain way, enough for a part within the subconscious... (now that's NOT the subconscious but rather a part *within* the subconscious) to go, "Yeah... got it." ... and the client sinks back to normality.

CHAPTER 3

Bob Hypnotises?

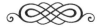

We're told that the universe is 13.8 billion years old. Our ancestors crawled out of the pool around six million years ago, whilst the modern form of humans only evolved about 200,000 years ago (civilization 'as we know it' is only about 6,000 years old). That would mean that we've only been here for .00004% of time. We're *new kids on the block* and most probably know very little about who or indeed what we really are. We've constructed this thing called science to keep us on the right path although many of our top scientists happily tell us that science is mainly wrong and continually being re-written. But I have to say in my own small way it's been fun discovering things about humans. Finding out that they're a little like belly buttons, 'all the same but just a little different'. Isaac Newton once said, "Finding out stuff is great, writing it down is secondary". But write it down I have. So... get the kettle on or uncork that bottle and buckle up...!!!

The hypnosis thing for me actually started back in 1973 when I was the lead vocalist with the band Cockney Haggis. Ray Chaston, the drummer in the band informed the duty manager of The Queen's Hotel, Aberdeen, as we were taking our gear in to set up, *"Don't look into his eyes, he's a hypnotist!"* I don't remember why he said it. We were simply loading our gear from the van into the gig where we were billed as, *'The Funkiest Band in Town'* ("I know...I know").

And she (Liz, I believe her name was) of course looked into my eyes. So... I simply told her to *"sleep"*, and I just caught her as her head was about to hit the floor (a couple life lessons learned in less than ten seconds)! Hypnotists reading the above will giggle of course (albeit a few will not be happy with me revealing that such an episode *can* take place) in the knowledge that the magic had indeed already happened in the mind of the young lady before I had even uttered a word. However, the very strongest investigator of this art will indeed posit the question: *Who hypnotised Elizabeth? Was it Bob who instructed her to sleep? Or was it Ray the drummer who informed her that Bob was a hypnotist? Or was it Elizabeth herself, who accepted the information from Ray that Bob was indeed a hypnotist before going on to obey Bob's instruction?*

Arguably hypnosis *can* begin the moment it's insinuated. To know that is to recognise its power. So, welcome to the world of hypnosis!

This event shook members of my band. They never knew I was a hypnotist. Neither did I of course, but wow, what a learning curve. But the shock of witnessing an induction (placing someone in hypnosis) never left me. Indeed today when giving workshops in hypnosis I would imagine that nearly all hypnotic trainers would agree that the students want to see inductions (preferably instant ones as this appears to be linked to some form of power perhaps, especially in men?) and I can understand this, although as a skilled therapists it is well down the scale of importance for most of us! But I reveal that wee story of my introduction into hypnosis for a reason.

And that is that many people believe, as I would have done, that hypnosis is something that we go off somewhere to learn from some wise man (or woman of course), far away from home. The truth is we, all of us, are capable of hypnosis at any given time. But of course, a working hypnotist will possess, and indeed practice their skills in nuance, hesitation, modulation, touch, feel, ambiance, strength, belief, intention.... as hypnosis is far more than just something which is taught. It *can* be of course, but it will be far stronger in the hands of someone possessing these very special arrows in order to fill their magical quiver. Yes, you can go to a hypnotist and learn skills but as Jon Chase wrote in his book 'Deeper & Deeper', *"I can teach you the skills, but you have to bring the talent".* Personally, like Jon, I'm not that sure if talent can be taught. Although if there is *something* there then of course it can be cultivated. I always used to ask myself, in any of the skills I had developed in any of my arts or disciplines, *"How sharp is my cutting edge?"* As you may know, a knife gets sharpened on a stone. Something as a butcher I know a fair bit about. But on top of that once you have your sharpened knife you have to *keep that edge on it.* And for that you need a good steel. Although a good knife man will sharpen his knife he also knows that just a couple strokes on his steel every so often will keep an edge on his knife all day, keeping it razor sharp and allowing it to do excellent work. And for me my steel is my therapy room. I'll just write that again if I may, *"My steel is my therapy room."* Sure, I can increase my knowledge by reading and conversing with my colleagues, but it is in the therapy room where we get to truly sharpen and keep the edge on these skills.

Nothing, but nothing, compares to a *practising therapist*. Right now we are bombarded on therapeutic forums with people claiming that this or that is evidence based (more of evidence based later), but it is in the therapy room where all the real evidence based work is discovered, with real people. I am often asked "What do you actually do? What can you fix? Who can you work with?" Several years ago, during one workshop for about 40 therapists, I said, *"It's funny, and I know a lot of you will want to strongly disagree with this, but recently I've come to the conclusion that nearly everything I deal with is actually: ANXIETY!"* And, to be fair, and indeed to my surprise not one person disagreed with me! I think good therapists come to realise that quite frankly, humans are anxious creatures. But they disguise that anxiety in many forms. WE should have a look at that though, shouldn't we...?

CHAPTER 4

It's an Anxious World

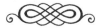

Anxiety is how a body naturally responds to any form of danger. When the person feels threatened, pressurised or facing a stressful situation an alarm bell goes off. Anxiety in itself doesn't have to be a bad thing in moderation. Indeed, it can be used to help one stay alert and focused or inspire one to act. It can even help solve problems. However, when it is ongoing to the point where it overwhelms a person, that can interfere with one's relationship and work to the extent that we can then be looking at an _anxiety disorder_. So, if we can agree that that's roughly _it,_ we can look shortly at how, in the amazing world of hypnotherapy, we can very often take a highly anxious individual and fix them in a very short period.

There are many studies of _anxiety_ being run continuously around the world and I wondered if you the reader would be interested in them and if so _how_ interested? e.g. would you want to read about how studies using functional magnetic resonance imaging (FMRI) which is used to learn how the brain functions in adolescents receiving fluoxetine (Prozac), cognitive behavioural therapy (CBT) or interpersonal therapy (IPT) for anxiety? Or how depression in children/adolescents works? Or perhaps the psychobiology of childhood temperament, which uses brain technology to examine brain changes that occur when children are exposed to various kinds of emotional tasks and to determine if these changes are related to the child's temperament. Or you might have a desire to examine the research which has shown that the corticotropin-releasing hormone (CRH) is involved in stress and anxiety, and how drugs that block the effect of CRH in the body can reduce that anxiety. Or you may want to read about the studies of *happiness*. Like the study from Tian Guoqiang (Shanghai University of Finance and Economics and Texas A&M University College), and Yang Liyan (Department of Economics, Cornell University Ithaca). A paper which studies the happiness-income paradox, revealing that as countries grow wealthier happiness levels do *not* increase. How their studies reveal that up to a critical income level which is positively related to non-material status, increasing income can indeed increase happiness, BUT... once that critical income is achieved, increasing that income further *cannot* increase happiness. In fact, somewhat surprisingly, social happiness is seen to actually *decrease*! Or you might have an interest in 'The Biology of Happy Emotions. Can a sunny outlook really mean fewer colds and less heart disease? Can enthusiasm, curiosity, hope, motivation, desire, love, laughter really protect against hypertension, diabetes or respiratory infections? *[as an aside I've just started feeling really happy as a strange coincidence has just occurred, 'Happy' by Pharrell Williams has just started to play in the background. And on Radio 4 to boot! Don't you just love serendipity?!]* Well, I have read and studied a fair bit on the above, much of it making my head go *boing*. And if you wish to look up the net it's all there for you.

They'll probably say it far better than I could, so good luck. But I *can* tell you about what I know and what I do. I work in a small room (sometimes there will be a third person in the room when I am mentoring). I light a candle, play some relaxing sounds (never whales or dolphins since a woman from Brechin complaining of anger attacks walked into my therapy room and pointed to the CD player exclaiming, *"And you can get that shit off for a fucking start!")*. Eventually there is a knock at the door and I say come in. They come in. I ask them to sit in *"the most hypnotic chair in the world"* and they do. Some giggle when I say this whilst others look at me as if I'm just a tad weird. I called this chapter: 'It's an Anxious World' for a reason. As I said in the last chapter I used to believe I dealt with lots of things in my therapy room, Smoking, weight, fear, phobias, OCD, insomnia, bulimia, dysmorphia etc. But I now believe that nearly all of my work (outside of chronic pain) is linked with people who are mainly *anxious* or that the thing they have is often developed through anxiety and I spend nearly all of my time working to make them *unanxious* in order that they can be happy. That's about it really. ☺ Believe me, I am under no illusion that I am someone with all the answers. This *stuff* did not come to me in a dream. There was never a burning bush (actually there have been several but they belong in a different chapter). Rather these have been my findings over many years. I was born in the 50's where most of us were brought up to believe that if we ever were given three wishes then we should always remember to ask for, *Health, Wealth* and *Happiness.*

I can even remember being told that health was far more important than wealth because *without your health you have nothing at all*. I guess there was always an assumption kicking around that if you had health and wealth then happiness would *have* to follow? Like a well-executed mathematical equation perhaps. I also remember how it all made perfect sense to me then, because the people telling me this were taller, older and therefore wiser than I. They knew things. They knew everything. Although I can also remember noticing how the taller older wiser people would often confuse me when, with this absolute knowledge, they would yet spend most of their time disagreeing with each other. But I handled that observation by doing what little people do, I totally suppressed it, telling myself that later, when I was taller and older and wiser, I'd have a look at why that was, maybe? But back to my small room. It is here I have noticed over many years how I get many exceptionally healthy people who flock to my door. I also receive many people of exceptionally high net worth. And to cut a long story short, other than the clients who come to see me with chronic pain, the vast majority of the time they will exhibit two things. The first is that there is anxiety within them (the male gender will sometimes even begrudgingly admit this). And the second is that they won't know (consciously) why this is. They will have ideas but in 99.9% of the time they will be wrong. That's why they come. Pondering over this 'Health, Wealth and Happiness' lesson given to me by big folks I can say that yes, of course I do get it, and it's not bad information at all. However, in the context of anxiety it really has no place.

[Thoughts to Steer By] So… in my work I have seen literally thousands of healthy people who are unhappy. And certainly, many extremely wealthy people who again were evidently devoid of any happiness whatsoever. The interesting thing is that I have never, ever, come across a happy person who was not happy. And as simple and obvious as that sounds, I want to bounce that off you just one more time, *I have never, ever, come across a happy person who was not happy.* And I felt many years ago that I should pay a lot of attention to that very simple truism. Having said that, in the therapy room when I ask, "What can I do for you today?" I have had several people over the years say, "I just want to be happy". When that happens I reach forward and tickle them under the *oxter* (word in Scotland and Northern England for *armpit,* Didn't I say this book would be educational?), then I ask, "Is there anything else you wanted today, or is that it?" Therapy then begins. I kinda' like people who come to me with anxiety. I *get* them. Many times, their stories are so perfect I want to cross the room and share the chair with them. I mean they know that they are stuck to a rock spinning round and round and moving through space at a squillion miles an hour (a rough model), and unless they get involved in an accident they will most likely have a stroke, contract a heart condition, cancer or malignant growth and even at the present time they are, at best, most definitely terminally ill, since death is indeed inevitable. Then there's the fact that many of them have embraced the universal truth that they/me/you/we are *never in control*.

Bad things will happen to them and/or their families (*this book will definitely lighten up later, I promise!*) so... they are anxious. And having mere money or stuff or even being ridiculously physically healthy doesn't do it for many of them. Nothing can, other than *a thought.* And that's what we do as clinical hypnotists. We get people to think a certain way, and their world becomes better.

Client quote (suffering from anxiety), *"My wealth hardly helps. It's strange but the Ferrari merely became the car after a couple of weeks and the mansion simply became a home in such a short time."*

I know that 'What is the purpose of Life?' is a huge question which has been asked for thousands of years. But what if the Prime Objective is, 'To be happy'? Does that mean that everything else just becomes, *narrative?* So... what is the problem for this anxiety? Is it simply that humans are an anxious species? And how do we fix it? *[....yes I do understand my existentialist buddies claiming that there is no Prime Objective and there's nothing to fix because there's nothing to BE fixed, it's all chaotic, but I find my clients need a wee bit more than that?]*

Yep, how do we fix it? Here we go... when you get involved in hypnotic discourse (especially in the world of Facebook forums) you will most likely be told by some therapists that nearly every protocol and practice absolutely works and with almost every ailment. And strangely enough, that doesn't have to be too far from the truth! Hypnosis is a truly phenomenal tool in the hands of a skilled proponent.

And a talented therapist should indeed be able to work with just about *any* tool. Indeed I suggested in an interview recently that rather than argue which hypnotic methods were best, I could take 10 of the finest therapists I know and give them tools which they were not *au fait* with and expect them to get great results! And that would be based on their rapport, their style, their activity knowledge, their know-how and of course… their *art!* For let there be no mistake, hypnosis is indeed an art. Something that many in so-called 'evidence-based medicine' simply do not realise. There is of course a good argument in knowing the cause of an effect in all forms of therapy, whether that be allopathic or alternative, however in the world of clinical hypnosis the experienced tried and tested therapists know that he/she does not *need* to necessarily *know* what the cause is. I can hear *some* of those who do analysis (where cause is imperative) screaming at me as I write this, but they're wrong and it might be a good idea to find out why they're wrong.

Remember I don't know the experience or knowledge possessed at this time by you the reader, but I feel at this point in time it might be a good idea to have a look at this thing called 'Hypno-Analysis' in order that we can get it out of the way? So, from the world of the analyst, and in particular the hypno-analyst there has been for many years a belief that all phobias are caused in childhood and in *most* cases under 4 years old. The next part, which was strongly believed for many years, and still is by many free-association therapists (but mainly Freudian analysists), is that the cause will be of a sexual nature.

Yes, I can see many other therapists shaking their heads at reading this but I have indeed met experienced therapists who have informed me that 'every single case of regression they have ever cured'... was indeed of a sexual nature and cured by evoking an abreaction, or what they sometimes term as, *'the bursting of the bubble'* (more of that in a moment). Now a free-association therapist will do their work by *placing* their client into an area or time: *"You are 3 years old and having an incredibly happy time. Where are you? Who are you with? What are you doing?"* However, it is important to understand that they try never to actually *lead* the client. Many modern-day therapists do try to make it clear that they are indeed free-association therapists rather than purely Freudian therapists (free-association psychoanalysis being a Freudian concept) arguing simply that they do indeed allow the client to free-associate more during the sessions.

Freud had what he would refer to as a, 'Fundamental Rule', where he would instruct the client, *"Never forget that you have promised to be absolutely honest, and never leave anything out because, for some reason or other, it is unpleasant to tell it."* I do know that some therapists find that slightly distasteful. Almost of a bullying nature? I myself have witnessed one session where I felt that the therapist was indeed putting words into the client's mouth in a way that was *beyond* leading (and told them so of course! We don't talk anymore.). But, that said, we are left with this very important belief which states (from the world of hypno-analysis, using free-association therapy) that the cause of phobias will have occurred under the age of 4 and be of a sexual nature.

However, I should very quickly explain that that sexual nature I speak of might not have actually taken place! Confusing huh? Well, welcome to the world of hypno-analysis, and since I often do get asked for my views on this very complex form of therapy, maybe we should spend a little time on a case study which indeed did take place in my therapy room, many years ago when I used to work almost purely as a 'hypno-analyst', which hopefully might explain this particular phenomena.

Case Study 2 (Hypno-Analysis)
Eve was a 37-year-old woman with arachnophobia (fear of spiders). She also suffered from the social anxiety disorder called ochlophobia, which is a fear of crowds. Eve was mainly anxious about walking into crowded rooms. Nobody really knows exactly why this happens however I can say that I have met many public figures of stage and screen who seem to be in control yet possess this same challenge. Eve informed me she had been fine most of her life, but these problems had both started around her 35th birthday completely out of the blue. I should say that in order to do analysis a patient does not have to be a great hypnotee. But they have to be able to relax, and simply say what they see, experience and indeed feel. Indeed, what they feel is the most important to the therapist. The following is from session 5. I spent only 6 sessions with this client. The last one more of a 'tidy-up' session, ensuring she was indeed cured (cured is not a word we use too often but I think when someone who had a fear of spiders is now giggling as a spider runs over their hand we're in fairly safe waters).

In Eve's case she went into a relaxed state very quickly and at my request easily travelled back through her twenties, teens, primary school to a time of pre-school where I asked her one simple question. At this point in time it should be explained that the therapist might ask the patient to go back to a time where they experienced pure happiness, surprise, laughter, pain, fear etc and await the response. They are asked who they are with, what they are doing, what's happening next. There can be lots of prompting and pacing but very little leading. And as said a moment ago, it's more important what they feel rather than what's actually happening. In Eve's case I had taken her through happiness, pain, fear, laughter and now I asked her to summon up the memory of herself as a child at a time where she felt loneliness. Eve had told of a time that she was in her parent's home. It was a Saturday night party for family and friends which would have been very common in working class Britain in the early 50's when Eve was at this age. She felt she was around four years old. She had earlier heard her mother talking to friends downstairs in the living room about how wonderful her older sister Amie was. Her mother hadn't mentioned Eve, only Amie. In the mind of this four-year-old there would have been no contextual thought. No understanding that someone could have asked specifically about Amie who may have been ill or going through a bad time at school and her mother had simply responded to that particular question. Eve only heard her mother talk of how wonderful her sister was, without mentioning Eve. In the therapy room when asked where she was now, she said that she was in the upstairs toilet, feeling lonely. When asked what happened next, she mentioned the noise of feet on the stair and how she had backed against the wall. Suddenly the door opened and there stood Mr. Daniels, a neighbour from two doors away. Eve likes Mr Daniels. "He's ran into the room and taken out his willie (Eve's words) and began to pee in the toilet." Suddenly he turns to his right and sees Eve for the first time. He acknowledges her with a smile and says, "Hello my wee darling, what are you doing up at this time, eh?" Eve went on to convey that although she had felt a form of loneliness prior to Mr Daniels entering the room she had then felt excitement. She could not explain the excitement but enjoyed the attention from Mr Daniel's and had indeed felt some other form of excitement when he was urinating. So, here we have the following situation, the 4-year-old child did not know what sex was and indeed was not feeling sexual. In this case we can fairly assume that poor Mr Daniels had ran into the toilet, started to urinate, then saw the girl. Eve then said that Mr Daniels (probably on realising fully the situation) turned slightly away and zipped himself up quickly. Eve also recalled that "he stopped smiling and looked angry". This was the words of a very confused 4-year-old girl. It might very probably be that Mr Daniels, on realising the potential assumed danger of what was happening was in fact not angry but looking concerned and wished to extricate himself from the situation. The next part becomes extremely interesting for a therapist, Eve had communicated her excitement. That excitement was due to the fact that instead of being lonely and feeling lesser than her sister Amie, she was now being given attention and she was witnessing the revelation of Mr Daniel's penis. This next part has to be fully understood.... Eve was not going through an actual sexual experience; however, she was looking at something she would have perhaps believed she 'should not be looking at'. She was in a situation she should not be in. And she was experiencing an emotion that she would argue (very quickly in her mind) that she perhaps should not be feeling. Even when Mr Daniels smiled at her (the poor man may have been mildly drunk at the time and not quite realised the situation for a few moments?) that felt good, perhaps being followed by a feeling, a huge dopamine rush. But then, suddenly a different feeling, perhaps supported by what she believed was his anger (he turned quickly and zipped himself up suggesting this wasn't quite right)? That was not good. Yet she had received comfort, a smile and seen something that she might have found different enough to appear exciting, if only in the sense that it was something that a part of her felt that 'she should not be seeing'. So, if you will, a form of pleasure but linked with that old favourite of the psychoanalyst, guilt. A guilty pleasure. Now that's 'guilt, real or imagined'. So, what does the mind of this child do in order to survive the situation? Strangely enough this assumed bad feeling which we might wish to term as guilt (real or imagined remember!) forces the young individual to do the only thing they can do with this fascinating mind they possess. Eve simply represses it (unconsciously). Her unconscious places it somewhere where she does not have to think about it, deep in her subconscious, where it stays, for a little over 30 years, until suddenly this young woman develops a total and complete irrational fear of spiders and a fear of people in a room. And then she finds herself in a therapy room, being regressed to the time of the incident, mainly through her own memories, until we find that one moment, the moment we were looking for. And the fascinating thing is that once that moment gets rediscovered and faced it simply explodes. It's not a four-year-old child that's in the room anymore, but a worldly 37-year-old adult who understands perfectly that this child is totally and completely innocent of any wrongdoing or guilt. Many times an abreaction involves tears initially but immediately after as here in Eve's case, those tears stopped (in less than 30 seconds) and Eve opened her eyes, actually smiled, then when asked, she answered that yes, she had indeed now a full memory of that incident. And yes, she can indeed confirm that everything the four-year-old Eve spoke of during the regression was in fact absolutely true. She totally remembers the whole incident and in this case, she actually throws her head back and laughs. And of course, we can report that no actual sexual incident even took place. Indeed, Mr Daniels was more traumatised than the four-year-old! Although he may well have been drunk and would never remember it again. Unless of course he might be in another part of the country right now, lying on a couch, talking to a therapist about his phobia! Let's unpick this case study just a tad further... - Now this is the part that some student therapists find difficult to understand. If an incident of wrong doing *had* actually occurred, strangely enough the effect might be *exactly* the same, and after the abreaction (abnormal reaction of a memory of the incident and feelings attached to it) the victim can indeed actually look back and simply let it go. And that's because the incident is *not about what happened. Not* about the act of the perpetrator. That did *not* cause the repressed memory of the incident. Rather it was a *feeling of guilt* (either real or in some misunderstood form) by the young person. And the reason why we know this? Because they *tell* us so! Time and time again. Isn't the mind strange? It's truly fascinating to talk to many men and women who have come through analysis, nearly all telling the same story of how, when the suppression was found, the abreaction took place (crying followed by clearance). Or as I said earlier, *the bursting of the bubble*. Here below is a diagram that might begin to explain what repressed memories might seem like in the human mind.

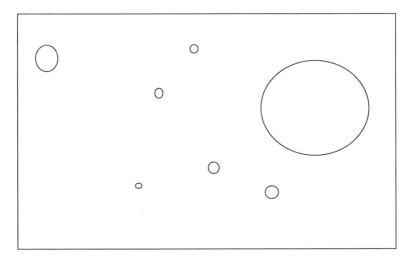

So, if you were to look at the mind as if it were in the above diagram, and if it were possible to assume repressions (every time anything was so bad they *cannot* handle it the person

Simply places/represses it way down deep into their subconscious), they might look something like these small bubbles. As you can see, some fairly tiny ones of things that happened and were repressed over the years. You can bet that we'll certainly hit that one (several repressions may be released during a session) at 11 o'clock on the diagram on the way to the largest one (the episode with Mr Daniels which caused the repression to begin with) hence a box of tissues is a must in analytical therapy, but… it's the big one the analyst is going for. Here you can see where the idea of the therapist finding the repression and presenting it to the client whereby an abreaction takes place is often called in analysis 'bursting the bubble'. However, whilst many of the hypno-analysts will argue that the *only way* to get rid of a repression is through analysis, which finds that moment in time and releases it through an abreaction, which in turn releases the memory (real or imagined) which then fixes the phobia, there are indeed many other ways. The skilled therapist will indeed hold many different types of methods in order to treat his/her patients and over the years they may change the main methods which they use. However, they will all favour one particular path, just as I most certainly do. And we'll get to that in good time. Can I just say that having worked as a hypno-analyst for many years I rarely use it now. Sure, it can work, but for me I found that there can be other much faster ways in dealing with certain clients. And, to be honest, I found that in doing analysis I was finding out things about the client that in many cases were *not relevant* to their particular complaint or phobia and I did not really need to know some of these very private intimate things. However, it is important to understand that when a person enters into therapy, they will indeed suddenly find a desire, with no prompting whatsoever, to tell their therapist almost everything about their life. It is a fascinating phenomenon to watch. So... let's look at *anxiety* in its very simplest form and in a way, it can be explained fairly easily. Anxiety is how a body naturally responds to any form of danger or worry. When the person feels threatened, pressurised or facing a stressful situation an alarm bell goes off. Anxiety in itself doesn't have to be a bad thing in moderation. Indeed, it can be used to help one stay alert and focused or inspire one to act. It can even help solve problems. However, when it is ongoing to the point where it overwhelms a person, that can interfere with one's relationship and work to the extent that we can then be looking at an *anxiety disorder*. So, if we can agree that that's roughly *it,* we can look shortly at how, in the amazing world of hypnotherapy, where we can very often take a highly anxious individual and fix them in a very short period.

Very quickly I should state that there are some very special therapists out there who claim they fix all of their anxious clients in one session and they are fixed for life. Indeed, many claim they do this in only ten minutes or less. And it's not just anxiety, it's everything. So let me just address this if I may. Yes both I and many of my trusted colleagues have had the luck and the wonder, and still do, to have these wonderful moments where we spend a little time with someone and they genuinely do, quite simply, just get...fixed. And it's instant. It can happen every week in our therapy rooms.

But the thing is there is no one person in the history of the world who has ever done this with their entire client bank. And if you should ever meet anyone who says they do (and I promise you there are lots of them) then you simply must...run away as fast as you can.

There, that wasn't so bad now was it? And so, it is I believe with all people who claim they 'fix people in one session'. It's not that they say it that makes me laugh. It's how when they say it, they pause, awaiting the world to applaud them, totally oblivious to the fact that those who understand therapy consider them to be not just riddled with their own hubris but highly thick individuals (Oh oh, looks like I'm off again!).

I have access to one million pounds sterling for anyone who can demonstrate their skills of fixing **everyone** in one session. Indeed, the offer was made in 2018 and linked to chronic pain. A wealthy friend of mine made the offer twice on my therapy forum (Bob Burns Hypnotherapy) and several people showed an interest, But when we got to talking contracts and they realised that you don't just turn up and 'have a go' (nobody gets offered a million bucks to have a go), but rather 6 clients would be chosen for you and your results checked over the next couple months, and good or bad these results would be revealed to the world, all the applicants changed their minds. Two of them cheekily claiming it was a false offer. Kinda' like Trumpian fake news! But the truth was when they realised that their success OR failure would indeed be reported they faded away.

For the record at this time of writing I work with my clients on an average of 4 sessions and I think I'd consider myself to be a decent therapist. I do fix people in one session (I won't be drawn into whether the therapist or the client themselves fix the problem as it's fairly long-winded) but I never DO only one session (unless it's a phobia such as fear of flying and they simply get fixed there and then). I always do a minimum of 2 sessions because I need to check my work. I am interested in *them*, in how they are!!! But I do indeed have clients who have been coming to see me for years! There's nothing actually wrong with them. I've told them so and they agree. However, they come in for 'top-ups' as they enjoy the sessions.

However, I would have to say the method I and many other hypnotherapists from around the world have used in preference to pure **Hypnotic Suggestion** would be **Parts Therapy**, and if you ask them why, I believe they will undoubtedly say because Parts Therapy can *fix* certain anxieties, rather than helping short term. And prior to discovering **The Swan** I used this excellent method for many years. Pioneered by **Charles Tebbits** it is a method of using hypnosis in order to identify and communicate with parts within a person's subconscious. The goal of course is to achieve a 'coming together' of the various (conflicting) parts within that person's personality in order to achieve cohesion. It is a beautiful teaching and therapy which Tebbits may have taken from the **Psychosynthesis Approach** of **Roberto Assagioli MD**. I do believe it would be totally wrong for me to even consider teaching any of the technical aspects of this wonderful protocol in this book. Rather I would strongly recommend the books and teachings of one of my colleagues, **Roy Hunter,** who I believe is the accepted proponent of Parts

Therapy in the world today. I have met many people around the world who have sat in on his lectures and workshops and I have never heard anything other than high praise indeed for this world class teacher. However, perhaps I might very lightly give an example that although is indeed simple I believe explains perfectly how the miracle of Parts Therapy works for anxiety, and seriously just about everything else. And we'll keep this ridiculously uncomplicated so that if you have a 7 year-old child THEY too would understand Parts Therapy!

Analogy of Parts Therapy

Imagine the problem, Mike Bruce the MD of Bruce and Sons sawmill in Diddlesbury, is receiving complaints from the girls in the office that the computers are sticking. Eddie, a local computer engineer, has checked the computers and told Mike that it would appear there's actually dust in the pads (technical term), indeed very fine sawdust. Mike pulls in Brenda, his office manager and Brenda thinks, then smiles, then tells Mike her theory. Mike is amazed, but realises Brenda is probably correct, because female office managers know shit! They now believe that the culprit is old Jim, who began working for Mike's father before Mike was even born. Every night old Jim takes care that the sawmill's main shed, next door to the offices, is totally swept clean. And they both agree that yes, it is indeed the work of old Jim that is causing this problem. The question for Mike is how to handle this delicate situation. He remembers what happened when his father told a much younger Jim 30 years ago that there would be no more smoking in the sawmill or indeed when they told Jim when his annual holidays would be. Jim went wild, contacting the union and the other guys who stopped working and all hell broke loose, until Mr Bruce stopped his authoritative manner, became more permissive in building a smoking shed and organising a holiday rota which _all of the workers agreed to_ and all the problems ended magically. And so, Mike pulls Jim into the main office. Gives him a cup of tea and a piece of Victoria sponge cake. Thanks him profusely for the past 50 years work, reminds him how _he_ has been of great help to Bruce and Sons over all those years, mentions lightly the past challenges but how _they collectively_ overcame them and then… asks for Jim's help. Jim asks what the problem is and Mike cleverly makes it very clear that, he totally and completely understands what Jim's actions are with a view to helping everyone working at the sawmill, as he has always done. Because THAT is what Jim DOES. However, it has recently been brought to his attention that in sweeping up the sawdust every night the dust is entering the computers… _"which we never had in the earlier days Jim so it's not your fault"…_ And so in not blaming Jim at all, but rather giving him this information, Jim has a think and comes up with ideas along with Mike, of brushing the sawdust another way, damping the sawdust down or even power hoovering the sawdust which they both LOVE and agree upon and Mike orders a power-hoover which arrives that same day. The funny thing is that while the dust in the computers stops and old Jim has more time on his hands, he even offers to give more help for the girls in the office with the mail etc.

Everything goes not just back together but gets even better!

And so through this analogy, here we see an important part within the subconscious (*Jim who is an important part of the sawmill*) unknowingly, creating a problem, until the problem gets pointed out and that part gets asked to change and even help. Perhaps even itself benefitting from the action in the fashion of *quid pro quo!*

Welcome to Parts Therapy. ☺

But, of course there is no therapy that works all of the time and sometimes we have to do something just a little bit different...

Case Study 3

I do remember probably the longest case I ever worked on where I was working with a young man who was severely anxious and suffering from body dysmorphia (or body dysmorphic disorder) whereby the person (very often females in mid to late teens or early twenties) is obsessed by some aspect of their appearance which they believe is seriously flawed. Quite simply he believed he was ugly and that everyone was aware of this and continuing to talk behind his back. Yet strangely enough he was indeed a handsome young man. The thing was he was not a good hypnotee (at that time) and in session eleven (that's right ELEVEN!) he got quite emotional, telling me he wasn't just crying because I couldn't fix him, but rather it was because I was his last hope. And when I decided I couldn't work with him (he felt himself we were close to that) he would have nowhere else to go.

In times like these you only have the moment. You don't have thinking time. A statement has been made by someone in severe anguish and they are looking directly at you, awaiting your answer. I could hear the clock ticking in my therapy room. It was my turn to speak and I had nothing to give him. But suddenly my mouth opened and I heard myself say, "Well look, don't worry about it, why don't you just keep coming back every week at this time. Don't ever bring any money, we'll just have some fun and we'll just grow old together. All I want you to do right now is lie back close your eyes and listen to the timbre of my voice."

After a couple minutes he asked me if he could open his eyes. Then he told me, "I'm actually feeling quite good!" That was it. He was fixed in less than a few minutes. I truly believe it was as though this part deep inside his subconscious was simply horrified at my response, it was as though the part thought, "What? Don't worry? Keep coming back? Forget the money? We'll just grow old together???!!!..... FUCK OFF!!!!!!" And it ran out of the room!

Several months later I attended his wedding. I gave him a full-length mirror as a present… for the obvious reasons! ☺ To this day, this client is now an excellent hypnotee and… a pretty good hypnotherapist!

So here we see that anxiety, like most ailments can be aided and indeed fixed (sometimes) by a mere suggestion.

CHAPTER 5

THE SWAN

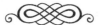

Very briefly you will recall in the chapter on anxiety I touched lightly on Parts Therapy. Again, if I can keep it simple Parts Therapy believes that 'the parts' are only within a person's subconscious, the goal being to generate a *coming together* in order to create positive change. But these parts are *not* real. Of course not! They are not separate entities outside the person themselves. That would be crazy wouldn't it? Anyway.... Welcome to The Swan. Are you ready? Are you sure?

There are many truly great therapeutic protocols in this world. These protocols carry a great deal of thought, having been constructed superbly by great therapists. They all carry an element of planning. Of Skill. Of wisdom perhaps.

BUT.... The Swan is devoid of any of the above. It took no thought. No intellect. No wisdom. No planning in any way shape or form. Quite simply it was a *happening*. It simply landed in my wee cottage in Montrose one Saturday morning. It could have landed anywhere and with any other person. It simply came along and said, "Can you see me?" That is about the best way I can describe its arrival. If I'm being candid, and I do feel I have to be, then I have to describe it as that.

There, I've said it. Phew! I'd love to think it chose me, and maybe it did! But I am very aware that there are many who Swan *better* than me and many now know as much as me about the protocol. I have to continuously remind myself (and I promise you I do) that whenever I am having an intellectual argument on what The Swan *is* or what The Swan can *do* I have to remember that just because I named this thing it does NOT follow that I know more than the next person with regard to what it actually *is*. Only that I do indeed carry specific thoughts on it, and yes, I am one of the most experienced people in the world in its use. I *do* use it Monday through to Friday every week and have indeed witnessed some amazing things, including some interesting characters, real or imagined, coming through the clients as they sit there, with maybe a sore leg, speaking to me in a language that they don't even understand. Let's just say the job is never boring. The great thing about The Swan is that it's most probably the only thing in the world that doesn't need to be sold! By that I mean that all over the world I walk into a room on a Saturday morning and see strangers staring at me. It's not so bad now due to technology since most of them now know, or *feel* they know who I am. They are, again thanks to the internet, au fait with The Swan. But in the early days there would just be me and the strangers. I would ask for a volunteer. They would come forward. I would claim to be about to talk, not to their subconscious, but rather a, part/energy/entity/angel/past life/guide/thing, *real or imagined, within* their subconscious. They must not try to fight me, and absolutely not try to help me. Simply allow me to do my work.

Basically, to allow anything that wants to happen… to happen. I would totally be aware that some people in the room (they'd even openly tell me later) thought I was an idiot. However, in less than two minutes, they'd be totally amazed at what they had witnessed when I did it with *them*, in many cases (again they would openly tell me later) their whole worlds would change. And of course, at that time, my audience has no idea that I am about to introduce them to another phenomena of The Swan; **Direct Voice**. Understand that some people on hearing direct voice for the first time have left the room… seriously! So, I hope you get what I'm saying here. That rather than me showing them how wonderful *I* am and/or making any claims to *my* skill…. I get to reveal to my fellow humans just how utterly amazing *they* are. And when I step back and let *them* do it, magic happens. Smiles, giggles, outrageous laughter, tears, F bombs being dropped… it all takes place when The Swan flaps her wings! And y'know what? Every Swanner in the world reading this right now is smiling, nodding their head and whispering *"yeah"*. Because that's what they have *witnessed*. That's what they *do*. They're Swanners! There's no inventor selling snake oil here or promising something that is highly exaggerated or doesn't quite work to the extent of what is claimed.

The Swan DELIVERS and in Spades ☺

As I said earlier in the book The Swan is now used by therapists, psychologists and indeed healers in well over 85 countries around the world and the feedback I have received, especially over the last 7 years (at this time of writing) has been truly wonderful.

I'd like to take a moment here to personally thank *profusely* all those fantastic people who have contacted me telling of their many fascinating stories of wonderful sessions and mind-blowing cures (which we will read about in another chapter) caused by *their* ability to use this simple protocol, attaching it to their own finely honed favoured therapies and skills.

Of course, it must fall on me now to spend some time on The Swan. Perhaps how it was discovered, developed, hated initially by a few and then loved and accepted by so many..... I remember having just returned from doing a couple sets of Tai Chi down in Montrose beach. It was a Saturday morning and I was sitting in my wee white-washed cottage in Montrose. My wife Leigh, a stunningly attractive and intelligent woman, was upstairs doing things that stunningly attractive intelligent women do in wee whitewashed cottages in Montrose on a Saturday morning *(I'm not being funny but I'm enjoying the style of writing I am bringing to this story!)*.

I was watching James Martin's *Saturday Kitchen Live* on the TV and I do remember my mind wandering as I started thinking about a particular client the day before who had found the therapy room and indeed the thought of hypnosis itself quite challenging. I guess it had been the whole thing about him already suffering from anxiety before he got there. And then finding himself in a small room with a stranger. The stranger is a hypnotist. He is about to be hypnotised by the stranger. The stranger will be in charge, and ultimately, the man, who feels already that he is not in control of his world, will be in less control. In fact, may be totally out of control!

All hypnotherapists reading the above will be able to relate instantly BUT they will also be experienced in handling this. It's what we do.

Where was I? Ah yes, in the cottage watching the cooking show. And so, after thinking about that client from the day before, my mind then began to wander off to other clients over the years. And then I found myself thinking of other people I knew who had told me that they felt they'd never be comfortable putting themselves in that situation. A hypnotic situation. A... *hypnotic* situation. I do believe I actually sighed (although my wife tells me I groan a lot when I am thinking) and for no apparent reason I did that thing we often do when we think, I ran my right hand through my hair, and then turned my head to discover my right elbow resting on the side of my sofa. My arm was straight up, and my hand was hanging there, extremely limp wristed. So, there I was. Staring at my hand, hanging there. And I swear out of the blue came that saying, "Talk to the hand". And so, I did just that. I talked to my hand. I said something like, *"So, look at you, hanging there. You actually look almost like a Swan. And look at me, talking to you, as if you're real."*

Then I think I giggled a little before the hand actually twitched a little, which in turn made *me* twitch! It was one of those moments, something happens that is slightly out of sync. But of course, I then assured myself that the twitch was simply that, a coincidental twitch. But, I was aware that I was now smiling, and I guess I then had to roll with it, so, I went and asked, *"Do you think you could do that again? Maybe twitch a finger?Maybe if you could just...."* And before I could finish... that's exactly what happened.

My forefinger raised up and fell down again quickly! I can very easily recall the happening as if it were yesterday. I was quite amazed, in fact, as someone who has worked with ideo-motor responses (IMR's) for many years I am very aware of what they are and how they work, but I personally had never been a great subject to work on. If I ever did get a result, then it would have been by being extremely patient. Relaxing deeply and waiting for something to happen. But this had been strangely *very* fast. So, I asked again, *"Do you think you could lift that finger again?"* *Bang....* it happened! And so there I was, sitting alone with my finger twitching *on call.* So, as the finger moves, I giggle, I ask, the finger moves again and I giggle again. I truly was amazed. But I wanted more. So, I thought I'd ask a silly question. One that I felt would *not* work, *"So, do you think you could actually... look at me?"* And instantly, just as my sentence ended, the hand and arm spun around to face me directly!

I let some noise escape from my mouth before immediately trying to fathom out just what the hell was going on. I wasn't giggling anymore and to be candid I was probably more confused than amazed. And then for a reason I cannot explain I asked, *"Well, aren't you going to say hello?"* And, of course, the hand *nodded!* How bizarre! I was both sure it was *not* actually me whilst having to confess that surely it could only *be* me. Surely it had to be some form of an IMR. An amazing IMR but an IMR none the less. I mean… It simply *had to be!* This was what I did with *other* people. But not with me. *Not* with me! And then, I saw it. I noticed that as my hand and arm had turned toward my face my arm was now leaning toward me.

50

I remember feeling both happy that I had sussed it out but also dejected a little that the miraculous moment had been broken? It would seem that my hand and arm had merely *fallen, by pure coincidence* on my command? Maybe with a tad of an IMR thrown in? But certainly, I could see clearly that this is what *had to have* happened. And it was here that fate stepped in. All I had to do at that moment in time was laugh at myself and drop my hand, I guess. That would have done it. Simply smile and drop my hand before turning to enjoy my cooking programme on the TV and that would have been it. Perhaps I would have left The Swan for someone else to find. Then I would have *heard* about it later, thought it was rubbish or considered it to be some form of an IMR, but on hearing what others in my peer group said about it I too would have bought the Swan DVD, tried it, found it to be absolutely fantastic and happily used it forever on my clients, just as I do now. But that didn't happen. *I believe life is all about moments.* Special moments. And that's what happened. There is a line in Ernest Hemingway's 'For Whom the Bell Tolls' that says, *'Today is only one day in all the days that will ever be. But what will happen in all the other days that ever come can depend on what you do today'.* (in THIS moment!) And I completely believe that The Swan operates all around the therapeutic world because of *that* moment, where I asked the next question. I guess that in order to simply close the whole situation, just to end it completely, I simply challenged this.... *nothingness*. This thing that I was sure wasn't even there. So I opened my mouth and uttered, *"So then, if you are real, if you are other than me, then I guess you should be able to lift my*

whole arm straight up and turn it completely, back away from me to face the front once more. Do you think you could do that?"
And I think that's when the screaming started!
"Leigh! Leigh!.... Leigh!"
My wife came hurtling down the stairs.... (she'll probably never read this, but if she did, she would turn her head slowly and glower at me, before uttering, in a clipped kind of way, *"I... don't... hurtle!")*

Anyway, Leigh came hurtling down the stairs and I simply said something like: '*I know nothing is going to happen. But just watch and honestly tell me what you think…"*

And so, I did the whole thing again as I watched my hand and arm dance for me. Twitching, turning, nodding and returning to where it was, which of course would be the very earliest training I would use in explaining The Swan… as I knew it then. Leigh was great. It was kind of like she had always known I possessed a sense of humour, but luckily realised that that sense of humour was much better than this craziness I was performing. So, she realised that this was real. Or at least I was not lying. And her advice was to get to work immediately with clients that following week and see if it worked with anybody else. Alas at that time Leigh was *not* a Swanner. But we'll talk about that a little later ☺

The Swan started working immediately that Monday although I used my smile, nod of the head, shrugs etc to veil my fear and laughter to cloak the feebleness I felt as I didn't really have a clue as to what was actually going on at that time with my clients.

I remember thinking how many of these clients would be assuming that this was me. This was what I do. That I was totally in control. But in truth they would have no idea that in reality I was almost totally out of control and didn't have much idea as to how this could possibly be happening.

Again, I would tell my clients what I always tell them, *"Don't fight me but don't try to help me. Just allow me to do my work, okay? Remember, your job is to do nothing. Now tell me are you left-handed or right-handed?"* The whole concept in these early days being to get them to witness something which they might consider to be something miraculous. In the business of course we call this a *convincer*. And The Swan is probably the greatest convincer I have ever seen that *something ese* is going on. Human progress has always been about expanding our limits. And of course, our beliefs. The Swan completely does this.

Around that time, I had a visiting student by the name of Maris Zalitis. Maris stayed on in Montrose for a good while after I did the initial mentoring with him and he and I became firm friends. When Maris saw The Swan, he of course loved it and it was indeed his idea to kinda' bring it to the world. He was almost upset with me for not calling it: *The Bob Burns Swan* as opposed to *The Swan,* but I've always had slight challenges with the eponymous thing. Also, at that time Camilla Edborg came over from Sweden to see my work and I have happy memories of being with these two beautiful people in my cottage, talking hypnosis and cooking for them. Can you picture it? Sitting there eating good food whilst my wife *hurtles* (I mentioned the hurtling yeah?) around the table filling up glasses with Merlot?

Since then I have gone on to do workshops with Camilla in Sweden which of course was a complete joy. In fact, I did my first ever Swan workshop with Camilla in Malmo. The Swedes seemed to like it whilst I felt I kinda' scraped through. It's difficult presenting something over 2 days when you're not completely *au fait* with it yourself.

After Sweden I took the action of going online and talking about my Swan where I got destroyed by just about everyone. One of them was a Greek guy. A clinical psychologist in London. After kinda' hammering me (as I remember it) in this forum he invited me to come to London and *show* my work, which let's face it seemed fair, so I immediately agreed to do it. The funny thing is when I met The Greek Guy, I found him to be lovely, and really knowledgeable on all forms of therapy. And so, it was that **Felix Ekonomakis** and I became great friends and we've travelled to the other side of the world working together since then.

But like I said earlier; life is made up of moments. And while that statement seems like a nothingness it is indeed a little hinge. And *on little hinges swing big doors*. And that belief that *life is made up of moments* is for me a HUGE door.

So, I'd like to take you back to that moment. When I did that workshop in London for Felix Economakis. As I said it was only the second Swan Workshop I had ever done but I knew that in this room would be psychologists and doctors and I would know nobody, and if I'm being candid, I have never been more nervous.

But just as we were about to start there was a moment. Felix introduced me to a lovely young man called **Yiannis Andritsopoulos** who had just flown in that morning from Athens to attend my presentation and workshop.

Yiannis had seen me on the internet and got the message I was doing this workshop. But he had no experience whatsoever, never done therapy before and no idea how to hypnotise. I felt obliged to tell him the truth which was that I honestly felt that this was not for him. I felt it would go way over his head. He had already paid for his flight but I asked what his hotel was costing him and told him Felix and I would cover that so he could enjoy a couple days but he thanked me and explained he was staying with friends. But he had a think about it and said he still wanted to get involved, that he was a quick learner, yaddyaddyaddy (I think that's Greek?)

And here's the funny thing. In taking that moment, that decision to allow Yiannis to stay I later discovered that he was the star of the workshop. I watched him working with the others and could see he was totally in the moment of every moment and more so than anyone. And why not? Yiannis was the only person in the room with no bad habits. He knew nothing, so he couldn't make any mistakes. Rather Yiannis was an open vessel. He simply listened and watched and repeated. And he got great results. The energy around him was palpable. Indeed, the next month Yiannis came back to the UK where he stayed with me and my English wife for three days. Being mentored by me in my therapy room, where I taught him my Consultation and of course The Swan.

After that I gave him some ideas on how to achieve the qualifications required to gain the appropriate training certification which would allow him to qualify for the necessary insurance required to work as a therapist and gain the proper Greek legislation to work in Athens. And as I sit here writing this I am looking at the message he gave me around 2 years after that, which says, *"Thankyou Bob, today I am seeing my 401st client!!!!!!!!!!!"* (he actually wrote more explanation marks than that! ☺ A beautiful moment eh? But of course, Yiannis was responsible for another moment. For it was Yiannis who recorded the moment which has allowed my wife Leigh and I to travel all over this world with The Swan over many years now!

After I demonstrated The Swan that day one of the attendees, a Frenchman by the name of **Philippe Miras**, asked if I could 'do it with him' during the coffee break. I asked him what exactly he meant, because he was French, y'know? Anyway, he said, "The Swan" and I said, "Oh, well that's alright then." It's bizarre I know but Philippe, whom I now regard as a good friend has been using The Swan since that day. He is a doctor of dentistry and has even brought it into many of his teaching courses which of course is wonderful. But that day, during the coffee break when I demonstrated it for Philippe just on a one on one, Yiannis was walking past, and as he saw us, he pulled out his phone and filmed it. A decision made. To film or not to film. Another moment.

The funny thing is that it was not a great Swan session, it was very long. LOL. Anyway it went online and a couple people saw it. And Voila....

In a very short period thousands of people saw it and recognised something. I believe they recognised that it was not an enactment. It was too slow, Too un-camera friendly. Which suggested that *this shit was real!*

People started contacting me (I have simply no idea HOW!) and I was advised to make a DVD of The Swan. It ended up being a 32-minute film of I believe excellent quality by a friend called Chris Tomlinson of Spectrum Films. The total cost was exactly £1,000 and I wondered if it might be possible that one day I'd get the money back! We didn't market it rather we placed a story of it in a forum. But the thing was everybody, and I mean EVERYBODY bought it and loved it.....! And, we got our money back by that Thursday!.... Then ...it took off... winging its way to over 85 countries around the world!... without one marketing clip ever being made of it. Because I don't know how to.

But now, a few years later, I have literally hundreds upon hundreds of messages (a few I'll let you read at the end of this book) from many people around the world and from many therapists and alternative healers revealing their experiences to me about what has happened to them and/or clients/patients of theirs in using The Swan. And of course, many of the very best therapists contact me weekly exchanging its uses with me. But now I think I should be brave and jump off the fence and make some claims. These claims I make are simply based on viewing the empirical evidence which has been clearly laid before me and colleagues over these last few years (albeit I will also say that if not one person had agreed with me I would still be saying what I am about to say).

So, let's get this statement out of the way. The first time I said this I was totally laughed at. But now, any decent therapist who has worked and continues to work daily with The Swan and many top-class stage hypnotists will tell you this, *'The Swan is NOT hypnosis!'* That's right, I'll say it again, *'The Swan is NOT hypnosis!'*

So, let's talk about that. First of all, with The Swan there is no induction (hypnosis is not attempted). Indeed, when I *perform* it, I ask the person *not* to close their eyes (although some will want to as they say they can't bear to watch the hand turn!). I also tell them that if I get a hint that they are slipping into a trance (and yes, they can do, I'm very, very good y'know!) I will stop the protocol. So, I am stating clearly that The Swan is *not* hypnosis. I am also saying that The Swan *is* a direct contact with a part of the *subconscious* (sc). On top of that I am saying that hypnosis is not needed *ever* in order to talk with 'a part within the sc' which is always listening. And yes, I'm sure some will pull me up on the fact that I said that I *perform* The Swan. Of course, I perform The Swan! I perform everything in the therapy room. I consider myself to be an artist. Therefore, I am skilled in nuance, metaphor, analogy. But also, in the case of The Swan, and indeed every form of protocol there is the art of hesitation, modulation and emphasization. And yes, although it is not needed with The Swan, I will use pacing and leading. Can't be helped, it's how I myself was trained and I like it! BUT... it's not needed. You very often find that in many cases the only things that are needed with The Swan are:

1) Honest enquiry.

2) Good manners. (that's right, remember you are talking to something/someone that *thinks*, therefore, *is*. God bless Rene Descartes).

3) Patience. "Remember that the engines very often need time to rev up" (a line from *Felix Economakis*) Who would have thought that Descartes and Economakis would be mentioned in the same paragraph? Rene will be chuffed 😊!

So, if we go back to where their hand is in The Swan position and I begin to comment, explaining to the client what might be about to happen: *"So here's the deal. When you came through the door a few minutes ago I noticed that you didn't bring your manual with you. That is to say I have no idea how you work. And, I need to know how you work. So, in a moment, I'm going to attempt to access that manual. I'm going to start by talking to your subconscious, through that hand of yours. And I'm going to try and do this without any form of hypnosis at all, just to see what happens. Then, one of three things will happen. Either your hand will actually move in response to my questions. Or, your hand will not move but you will feel it wanting or trying to, or it is possible that your hand will not move and you will feel no sensations. Again, that's perfectly alright because once again I still regard any of that as feedback, a hint or at least an essence of how you work. Is that okay?"* I then demonstrate for them the shape of The Swan. Then I tell them I *don't* actually want that rigid shape, rather I want the hand to flop 'like this'... and I make my hand go limp revealing no rigidity. Then The Swan Protocol takes place.

Both **The Swan** and **The Swan Speaks** are, for me, far better demonstrated by visuals rather than described in writing, and so I strongly recommend that you the reader check out the downloads, which can be found in the shop on my website:

Bobburnshypnotherapy.com

However, keeping in line with the KISS principal (keep it simple stupid), The Swan is indeed this simple: Twitch, Turn. Wave, Return, that is all we are initially asking the hand to do. Then we might wish to ask how it would say yes and no to us. But... it IS that SIMPLE.

In closing I feel I need to point out that whilst I say that The Swan is neither hypnosis or IMR, I need to say that it can very much *move into being* both hypnosis and IMR. It's one of those things where, once you get experienced you watch this occur now and again and get it! Quite simply read what I say about IMR's in the chapter: 'The Consultation', where I explain IMR's through the use of The Pendulum. The Swan is *not* that. It *will* argue with you as you will witness in The Swan Speaks and indeed I have been told along with literally hundreds of my colleagues from around the world to *"Fuck off!"* many times through the mouth of the client during The Swan Protocol. No IMR's and no hypnosis. Just one highly embarrassed client 😊

I have already mentioned anxiety in clients. Probably THE biggest challenge I have personally found in people. It can cripple everything. And it is a fact that we can often find ourselves at the very beginning of every first consultation with a person who is a bit scared of hypnosis, and much of that time because they have a fear of losing control.

Here is how I would advise you handle it. Based on the magician's code that: **'If you can't hide it then paint it red'.** Said to client: *"A lot of hypnotherapists, are really, really nice, in telling you not to worry about losing control, because in this thing we call hypnosis you will be totally in control at all times. Isn't that lovely?"*

And they seem to like this. They seem to be happy. Then I 'knock them off their feet' (we'll explain knocking them off their feet later) by saying, *"… but why would you worry about losing control when you are already totally OUT of control? Now that's true isn't it?"*

This will prompt a slooooow nod as the realisation steps in. *"That's why you're here. But here's the good news. It's MY job to totally take control. And that's exactly what I'm going to do, for you. My goal is to take total control, clean up the entire problem and then when I've done that I'm going to hand it back to YOU, in order that you can then actually BE in total control and handle your life with relative ease. Does that make sense?"* The nod might be accompanied with a smile at this point. *"Then let's make a start, sorry did you say you're right or left-handed?"*

So yes, it is indeed my intention of *taking full control of the situation*, cleaning it up and then when it's fixed handing that control over to them.

In closing this little segment I did mention my English wife earlier. Leigh, remember? The hurtler? I also admitted that way back then on day one I got no response from her with regard to The Swan. However, some three years later, I was doing a workshop in Belgium with Rob de Groof (who now runs his own trainings over there and indeed we often bump into each other in many exotic places around the world). Rob had originally attended my training in Scotland before inviting me over there to do a workshop. I had finished the actual workshop for Rob, but I was now doing something a little different. It was I believe a Monday evening and the theme was, 'How to put the magic into hypnosis' and 'Magic with a hypnotic twist'. As you might imagine we had a full room consisting both of magicians and hypnotists. At one point I asked everyone to lift up their left hand. I can imagine at this point in the book that you the reader have been asking yourself about my English wife. How she must love what I do. An extremely attractive magical hypnotist! She must follow that man everywhere. Well the truth is that Leigh never ever comes to anything I do. She quite simply travels the world visiting art galleries and buying shoes and we meet up in the evenings for drinks where she shows me her shoes and pictures of art. It's... fantastic!!! Anyway, this was the only time in our lives where Leigh had nowhere else to go and had to attend the procedures. It was difficult for me also as I could clearly see her sitting in the middle of the audience, trying not to cry. I was so proud of her. Anyway, the fun part came when I did an audience Swan group demonstration. As Leigh's hand turned and nodded towards her face, I realised I had never loved her more. She was obviously only doing this for 'her man' (something she has always proudly called me, in her own way). We had arrived together. Everyone knew she was my wife. She obviously did not want to embarrass me by everyone seeing that my wife did not *do* The Swan.

That would have come across as a disaster! So, the evening ended and I *finally* got Rob de Groof to get a round of drinks in (one of my greatest international achievements!) before we called it a night. Then once back in our room I thanked Leigh for doing that. It was just a little white lie and nobody got harmed. And again, I felt the room grow cold. She gave me that eyeball to eyeball look as she once again did that clippy thing with her voice: *"Do you really think I would turn my hand for you? That thing had a mind of its own! It was going completely crazy!"*

So, the good news of course is that this was a fascinating convincer for Leigh and I can report that later that same evening and right up until today, although not a somnambulist Leigh does indeed have the ability to enter this place we call hypnosis very easily. Sometimes we need to simply wait for the special stuff. WE need to just take our time and enjoy the ride. I call it 'delayed gratification'. *Sure, the early bird gets the worm, but it's the second mouse that gets the cheese!* 😊

See chapter 13, page 186 (Swan cheat sheet)

CHAPTER 6
Scripts

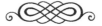

(The Importance and Development of)

Before we begin, I want to ask the script-haters reading this to allow me some leeway. Then you can judge my thoughts on this quite spicy topic. Is that fair?

Yes, I was absolutely on your side of the fence many years ago and YES...I will be using the word SCRIPT a lot...BUT... I would like you to allow me to reveal precisely what I mean by it, and if you can I'd like you to *not* see some paper with words on it, but rather a *'master template'*. Indeed I have to thank a former student and now fellow colleague, John Gotelee, for suggesting this synonym to me several years ago. And he was indeed correct in that many people uncomfortable with the word script are much happier to consider a template. So thankyou John. Now we can begin...

When I am delivering a workshop I like to begin by asking each attendee (allowing for time and dependent on numbers being not too high) to briefly introduce themselves, talking of their experience to date and perhaps mentioning the reason why they are here. Indeed, if they are brave enough, I ask them if there was one gift I could give or teach them over the next few days what would that be? It's a great question. All they have to do is be honest.

And the thing is that the majority of practicing therapists who either come to me for personal mentoring or attend any of my workshops around the world normally reveal (although of course there are others) one or the other or even both of these two challenges:

a) They lack a certain confidence in their personal abilities as a hypnotist or therapist.

b) They are not entirely happy with the *style or technique or process* of therapy they trained in and feel they need something more.

Those are by far the main challenges I am given by people attending my workshops. And it is for this reason that I teach others to use my very simple system in the therapy room, which I call, THE WALL (chapter 8), which is a scripted process, and when I am teaching live in the therapy room the student with me gets to witness this method being successfully used with every new client that walks into the therapy room. But I think it might be a good idea to go back in order to find out where The Wall came from, and for you to know *why*.

Stan the Man

I believe I can say that I am recognised by my peers around the world as being a fairly highly skilled hypnotist and therapist. And I truly believe that I owe all of that to the fact I was a highly skilled salesperson. Today I believe that a great therapist IS a great salesperson. And I became that because of being highly trained and by being given great advice from many mentors. One of the main ones being Stan Metheney.

In the eighties I was sitting on a train travelling towards Telford with Stan who was a very senior manager and trainer from New York Life, one of the biggest companies in the world who had just bought over Windsor Life, a life assurance and investment company in the UK. Each time they bought over a company New York Life would seek out the top sales executives and managers within that company and spend time dissecting them. Studying them for weeks. Finding out what they knew, how they operated, with view to incorporating their skills into the hive. So, I guess I was very honoured that I had been chosen to be shadowed by one of their very best men. However, Stan was in the middle of breaking the news to me that... I was not 'the one' ☹! He did say I was extremely gifted, but the problem was that all my talents seemed to be intrinsic. They were locked up in a mishmash inside my head. He informed me that I had some wonderful skills, BUT in reality, over the weeks chatting to me (in what seemed to me at the time like open discussion but evidently was *not*) he said he had discovered that I didn't seem to have a clue as to how I did what I did. That I was naturally talented as opposed to having transferrable skills (a problem with many trainers). I had no scripts, no formulas, nothing I could pass on in a way that would be understood by the execs back at the Home Office (American term), other than a few phrases I seemed to favour. He confessed that these phrases were indeed quite clever. He liked my nuances. my touch. my smile. my 'head-nods'. my eye contact and how I would shrug my shoulders and make open handed gestures when closing.

I never even knew I shrugged and made open-handed gestures and told him so. "I know" he exclaimed. "That's what I mean Bob. You don't know what you do."

I was disappointed that New York wasn't going to fly me over and toast me, but I clearly remember as Stan was revealing my lack of real knowledge, thinking to myself as I smiled into his face, *"Shit... he's right. I just act like I know what I'm doing and it seems to work out fine most of the time. But I don't really have a clue! In fact, I don't really recognise what he's saying as he describes me to myself."* Looking back, I suppose I did have a little bit of impostor syndrome. I wasn't quite *gallus* (Scottish word for 'cheeky self-confidence') enough.

Years later as a successful manager I remember interviewing a Glaswegian guy who said, *"Look buddy, I'll just be honest with you, there's no point in you asking me awe them technical question cos , I don't know shit, A'm only good at getting results!"* and I had him on a train to our training department that afternoon! People who truly *believe* they're good at getting results are normally, good at getting results! Stan went on to tell me I would keep winning awards and grow within this or any company I ever wished to work with. However, if I ever wanted to get into the very top in executive management or training and helping others, I would need to be able to both *learn and reveal* these skills I possessed to others. Because, he said: "You can never give others your talent. You can only teach them your skills (something I said in an earlier chapter). And you need to know exactly *what* these skills are and *where* you keep them."

So, he suggested I study myself and everything I know. So, let's see where we are. At *that* time, we have a decent sales consultant and middle manager with a small sales team. He doesn't really know how he achieves his results, yet he is a national award winner in both sales and management. But that's not completely true of course. Like all great salespeople I had been trained to be *'scripted on the pitch'*. I had luckily been trained by other great salespeople before me whom I had studied and I learned their words on presentation. I knew their interruption stoppers, their rebuttals, their soft and hard closes. Their switch sales and how to get a personal recommendation as opposed to a *mere* referral, and of course how to know the difference. But I wanted to be better. I'd have to have more words. I needed to record myself saying and doing what I said and did, and then write it down and study how best to teach these skills to others in order they could duplicate my results (*dictaphone was the hi-tech of the day back then*). I moved into and through the management ladder where I learned how to stop trying to *recruit* people but rather concentrate on *rejecting* them (a team builders' greatest skill). That way I'd get the *best* recruits. In fact, after a while I learned how to put my ego aside and started securing my recruits from people whom I considered were possibly better than me but in the need of some *tuning*. Then I'd train them whilst watching and learning from *them* (again something I still do to this day), where I discovered that the very best of humans are happy to share. Then of course I had to find a way to change some of the message slightly in order to find a way to teach it to others.

I'd watch someone using a skill which I would take apart and rebuild in such a way that I could explain their skills better than they themselves could. *I learned very quickly that the best way to teach someone something is to show them. Reveal* the authenticity of what you are saying. Make them smile as the revelation hits them so hard, they have an 'ahaa' moment!

First of all, I had to get *my* attitude right. I had to imagine that everyone I would train would be my best friend. That I would want to give them the very best of me. I was aware that the reason why I had become the top area manager in the past was that I was just about the only manager in the UK who physically went out with my reps and went into areas that required hard work and effort. I had even become aware that although I got on with other managers several of them knew that their sales teams had talked to members of my team and *knew* what I did and those other managers also knew that they themselves did not do what I did. They lectured and showed charts whilst I was taking my team *down the street* (*in* the field) and showing them how to help people and make money as a wonderful by-product. I went on to become the national sales manager and I knew stuff. Lots of stuff. AND I was pretty damned good at passing it on. I could literally tell a rep to *say this like that as they moved like so* and they would get a result... and they did! That's probably why I'm writing this book! So, cheers Stan ☺ *And little did I know that this is exactly how I would be mentoring professional hypnotists and hypnotherapists forty years into the future!*

As I said earlier, I mainly train people IN the therapy room in REAL time with REAL patients with REAL problems. I believe it's the very best way to train someone in therapy. Could you imagine working for over 10 years in allopathic medicine, desperately trying to become a heart or brain surgeon and then getting a certificate without ever having to step inside an operating theatre or seen any blood? Welcome to the world of hypnotherapy! You really couldn't write this stuff, could you? As therapists who train others, we don't need regulation, we just need to stop rehearsing in workshops and start taking people who are desperate to learn INTO our therapy rooms. That way they are in with at least a chance.

And when I take a trainee into my therapy room (even if it's a virtual therapy room online) I show them and teach them my scripted consultation. Scripted because as the wonderful actress Judy Allen once wrote,

"Nobody can give a good performance unless the authors and composers have written a good part for them!"

Important Disclaimer

Before we take another step, I want to make it clear that when I am working with an ongoing client over sessions, I do NOT use any form of script in any way shape or form. **The ONLY time I am scripted is in my Initial Consultation**… which is an area that I feel I need my cutting edge to be razor sharp. I want to dot all the I's and cross all the T's. I have no room for mistakes and I need to ensure that I have properly delivered a whole load of information and gained everything I need to from the client at that specific time. So, for me there is no room for error. If a client 2 years later were to say that I forgot to tell them so and so at the time of the consultation or that I had actually *said* a certain thing, I would know if that were true instantly! That is because I am so well scripted I know that every consultation I do it is totally impossible for me to make an error, forget something or to waffle (other than a fully controlled waffle and for a specific reason! 😊).

So now let's have a look at, **Pros and Cons of scripts**

First of all, can I just say that I have nothing against people who are not remotely interested in learning the skills of being a scripted professional. I was that person and I did just fine. I was talented. I had natural rapport. I was happy. But then I spent time with a guy watching him at work and I was totally blown away. He totally (here we go again) *went with the flow* (or rather *looked like* that's what he was doing) until by the time he did his third presentation that day I realised I was in the presence of a fully scripted professional. Oh, don't get me wrong, he could leave the script and come right back to it at any juncture he wished. He was that good. And so… I followed him, and I learned stuff that I never knew before, and I felt totally empowered, and still do to this day. What I am saying is that in my experience I can train a better therapist if I give them my skills and teach them how to use those skills, anyone can. But when I give them and train them how to use a good script their skill levels will totally explode! But here are the main **cons** I have heard in group conversations over the years on scripting:

You have to take time writing stuff down and learning it (yes, somebody actually said that LOL)

They make you sound robotic (this is a perfect description of someone demonstrating that they have not learned the work)

People can spot a scripted person a mile away (The exact opposite is true. They cannot. Not when it's a professional demonstrating that work)

A successful therapist never uses a script.

(non-script users can be successful of course. But this is said by someone with no idea of the subject)

It stops your flow

(although the exact opposite is true, I have heard from many therapists: "Personally I prefer to go with the flow" and when I ask them to demonstrate they turn into a lump of jelly. My findings have been that it is not their fault. Rather they have been insufficiently trained, meaning their cutting edge is blunt, thus they have challenges 'going with the flow'. Or rather they simply cannot flow.)

When you talk to a person who does not use a script or rather is not scripted (there is a difference of course which we will get into later) you get to hear them explaining why they don't actually understand scripts or being scripted. As said earlier, the funny thing is that every good therapist _is_ or _becomes_ scripted! i.e., they will have successful programmes of speech which they continually run (even when they don't know it!). But I'm saying that it's best to travel that road with _intention_. And of course, if we look at the cons, we get to recognise the positives, BECAUSE you have to write stuff down you are forced to think things through. Designing every single word with a purpose in mind. And in its use, you will discover real facts about what works and what doesn't work, and you will *know* these facts. Through this process you actually learn and remember your work.

With practice you sound as if you really do know what you're talking about. Nobody *ever* knows when a skilled person is using a script.

All successful therapists ARE scripted. It's just that many of them are not aware of it! And if they practiced, they would be even better! When shared with peers and colleagues you get amazing feedback and get to discover new things to add or make even better which over time makes that script almost perfect in getting its desired result, turning it into a genuine evidence-based practice. So YES…new things can be added and subtracted over time to sharpen its cutting edge.

In the world of sales (all great therapists SELL) it is recognised that anyone can have a bad moment or a bad day but with a professional scripted presentation it becomes literally impossible to have a bad week.

Strangely it has also been proven that scripted presenters are actually better listeners. And this is because they are so skilled in their presentation it is in-built right there in their subconscious, as it (the subconscious) drives the car, allowing you to enjoy the scenery. To 'take-in' the beauty of it all.

I guess what I'm saying is that scripted people possess a form of muscle memory which in itself, can really allow the user to *truly* 'go with the flow', as opposed to others who *think* they are doing that. In sales it is known as 'straight lining', taking you from *hello* to 'the close' whilst handling all challenges on the journey, because you know what those challenges are and how they can always be handled. Understand that there is nothing wrong with a highly trained therapist, knowing their profession inside out and allowing themselves to be totally at ease with every single person who steps into their therapy room as they use their finely honed and well-practiced protocols whilst they think of the best way to help their clients, built on their vast experience. BUT…they had to get there. And they probably did not get there by naturally 'going with the flow'. The very best of them knew what to say… at what times… and how to say it. The challenge with the average professional therapist today (2021) is that they see an average of 2 to 3 people per week and average an income of around seven thousand pounds (£7,000) less expenses (*These figures did NOT come to me in a dream! My friends and colleagues in Europe, Australia, America and Canada assure me their countries tell similar stories*). And the training rooms keep filling! Don't get me wrong, many of those therapists are indeed *excellent* in their work and I think it's a lovely thing that people are healing people, albeit in many cases in a part-time basis. However, for many of them that was never their goal. Rather they were sold a dream and a career (just like those sales reps of the 60's, 70's and 80's). They need to pay the mortgage and eat and I have found that staying alive and not going bankrupt is a great way of doing that.

And I know of several really good therapists who are now working at *something else* whilst we are surrounded with people who could use their help as opposed to being filled up with tablets. So... that's why I am not a lover of using one's assumed natural gifts in order to, 'go with the flow'. Remember what I said earlier, sure, if you're a trainer you can teach people your skills, but you will NOT be able to teach them your talent! Rather you will simply show them how clever YOU are, which is of no value to THEM. (Don't *read* scripts. Learn them) So let's have a look at this world of *being* scripted in the therapy room.

Can I just say that the lack of confidence in the beginning of one's career can destroy a therapist? To be honest in the very early days of therapy I have to confess that I simply *read* scripts (WRONG!)! The secret was to *seem* totally relaxed. Get the client to take a deep breath and close their eyes and..... as I rambled on, I would slide out my script, very slowly, and then of course try not to make too much noise when I slid a page away. You know the noise. When paper slides against paper. It sounds kinda' like sssssshhhhhhtttt. I used to be so nervous I would even believe it actually sounded like *shit*. I used to cough a lot so the client wouldn't hear the paper sliding! My earlier scripts were so bad they went like this, "…..that's right, all the way down until you find yourself totally relax… (shiiiiit-COUGH) …ing as you simply go deeper and deeper."

Jeez, but I used to panic so much as I turned those damned pages. But there it was in those days. I would read it to the client in the hope that this script in itself would fix them. And, lo and behold, several times it did just that! But I wasn't a therapist and I knew it.

The funny thing was that the words on the page were quite good, as is so often in scripts. BUT…I was *reading* the script. I might as well have sent my milkman to do the job! And I think that this is the main argument anti-scripters have… which I promise you I do GET! I totally understand what you are saying!

But in no time at all of course I realised that I should re-write my script into a generic script that might suit *all*, in order to get them to a certain place, where they can find themselves in a state of total relaxation, in order that I could then do my real work, which, after a few years was to quite simply *truly* be able to: 'go with the flow'. But just in case you haven't got it by now, the only time one can really go with the flow is when one *can* go with the flow knowing all the bases are covered. And I could go with the flow of course, because I was scripted. That is, I knew exactly what to say and when to say it…without having to hold a script in my hand. But it was the learning of the script that got me there.

So, let's see if I can clean all of this up. I am saying that in the early days, no matter how good a therapist might *think* they are they are probably not! That they have just passed their driving test which means they can *now* learn how to drive. And the best way they can learn how to do that is to be scripted. *NOT in the way where they are continually reading a piece of paper,* but rather that they are fully trained on order to get from A to B to C etc without the chance of making a *faux pas*. That they are totally and genuinely in control. Here is the analogy I use in every workshop I ever do; You are catching a train from Aberdeen to London.

You wish to leave at 9.00.a.m. and plan to arrive in Kings Cross, London at 4.35.p.m. Your route will be through Stonehaven, Dundee, Edinburgh, York etc ... and at any one of these stops you can alight from the train, spend the proper and allotted time buying a newspaper or a coke and then step back on. The good news is that simply by the train staying on the rails, and hitting every station on time it will be *guaranteed* to arrive in London on time *(please take the workings of British Rail into consideration at this point in time. I'm only bloody human!!! But hopefully you get my point?).*

When I was asked to learn scripts back in the 70's I promise you this was the exact analogy I was given by my mentors and I accepted it because it made sense. Others did not of course. They went with the flow... all the way out the door. So, I often hear how bad scripts are and how the person could spot one a mile away. Well, not when I use it, they don't. But remember I only use them to get me where I can then do my work. So please understand I am scripted from the client entering the door till I get to address their specific problem. *Then*...I *openly* flow. And I can leave the script anytime I want, remember just like leaving the train to buy a paper, then stepping back on and continuing to Kings Cross London, on time and guaranteed.

The secret of training oneself to read scripts lie in four words and here they are, *Practice, Practice, Practice, Forget.* And the lovely thing is you then find that because you paid that price of practice you find it impossible to forget your skill. But... you *have* to *pay* the *price*. That's the deal. You can have just about anything you want in this world as long as you do two teensy

77

weensy things. First you find out what the price is. Then you decide whether or not you want to pay the price. Of course, you don't have to. You can spend years in the wilderness telling everyone of how you just like to go with the flow.

Now I should say that every now and again when I am mentoring someone in the therapy room I shock the hell out of the student by getting the client to take a nice deep breath and close their eyes, then I actually, ...*slide out and read a script!* Just to show them (the student) I *can* and that it's still not a problem for me to do it even with all my experience. For I am The Author of everything that happens in my therapy room. Let's go off in a slight tangent...

The Elevator Pitch (in reality, 'a small script')...The first time I heard the term 'Elevator Pitch' I smiled broadly. I got it instantly. I already knew what the 'founding fathers' (Caruso and Rosenzweig) of that term meant and why, *and* I recognized its power.

At this point in time, since we are talking about scripts, I just thought it might seem remiss of me if I were to miss out something incredibly simple yet *so* important in the quiver of any therapist out there. Hopefully this won't insult anyone's intelligence but for the uninitiated here is an example. Imagine yourself in a scenario where you are in an elevator (*assume it's December, you'll find out why in a moment*). Let's make it a huge building owned by, 'Virgin Group' and you're about to undertake a 30 second journey in the elevator.

The door goes *ding* and as it opens in walks Richard Branson (*wearing a jumper with a Christmas tree on it*) He stubs his toe on the way in and exclaims, *"Fuck me!"* You absolutely do *not* move (it would quite simply be the wrong thing to do!). Then he looks up at you and says, "Sorry about that I'm Richard Branson. I've never seen you in here before. Can I ask what you do here?" (look it could happen right?). So, your job, within the next 30 seconds or less, is to grab his attention and interest. Here's the deal, If the best salesman in the world says, "I'm a salesman" Or the best artist in the world says, "I'm an artist" Or the best brain surgeon says, "I'm a surgeon" Richard will most probably smile politely and leave on the next *ding*. That's because they've just given Richard Branson a sausage. But Richard Branson does not buy sausages. Richard Branson buys *sizzles!* So, at the risk of making myself look a total *numpty*, here is just one of *my* elevator pitches:

"Hello Richard, My name is Bob Burns and I work with people all over the world, helping them and training others to deal with all forms, of worry, anxiety and stress in the workplace, which of course can cost companies like yours millions of pounds each year. I am well known for having developed a certain protocol that works for those types of people and I'd love to demonstrate it for you! Here's my business card."

So, in 73 words and less than 20 seconds I have hopefully sold Richard Branson, not a sausage, but rather a sizzle! I have grabbed his attention and interest. If my pitch is good enough (and I'm scripted remember? I'm professionally trained. I do NOT just, *'go with the flow'*)...

79

the conversation might now continue beyond the elevator ☺. Remember what I said just a few minute ago\? 'All hypnosis and therapy is about being a great salesperson'. When you get that part inside to nod its head in agreement with you, the fat lady sings her song (wow, that's deep yeah?..... Yeah?)

And because I believe that being a great therapist is about being a great salesperson and indeed mainly scripted I even take this belief into such minutia as presenting my business card. Yes I know. I know you're thinking 'old school' and who would present a business card in the modern world? And the answer is: someone who understands the power of a moment in the modern world (sigh!). C'mon guys keep up. So if I have nothing to lose by handing out my business card and everything to gain why would I not hand out my business card? Especially since I'm not just a normal person handing out a business card I'm *me*... Bob Burns. So buckle up, and learn how *you*... can *take* a moment in order to *make* a moment. A moment that will make the recipient remember you and what you did in that moment.

The Presentation of a Business Card.

So, when you give your business card to another human being a new contact is being established. Remember what I've been telling you... that *life is about moments,* and this is a moment, where you have an opportunity.

For me a business card should *never EVER* be given, it must always be *presented* in a way that makes the recipient remember you for the rest of their life.

(Although I had devised and used this idea myself the idea of printing the card came from one of my favourite magicians Michael Amarr) Let me show you what I mean.

So get online and look this up:

Clip 1 YouTube: How to present a business card

Let's move a back a little... I had now realised that Stan The Man was correct. That I needed to give the people I was responsible for even more. A map. A path. A kinda'... **script!** Something that would get them from A to Z. A big heavy stick which they could use to defend themselves long enough... until they had learned how to hone their skills in the style that they wished. So... I remember starting off by attempting to write what I thought was the perfect opening line. Something that was fairly universal. A track to run on that everyone could use with ease. An initial line leading to a script including, interruption stoppers, rebuttals, emphasisation (it's a word okay? It's a word!), modulation, explanation, throwing off, taking back, positivity, statements, smiles, (yes you need to know when best to smile and when *absolutely* not to!) pauses, direction changers, ahaa moments, head nods, closes etc in order to give the trainee executives all the time in the world they needed in order to allow them to allow *themselves*, that part within, to truly, go with the flow.

So just for the record, if I am boring some of you by what you consider to be me going over the top with this scripting thing and this 'going with the flow' phrase, then GREAT! That was and is totally my intention. It's totally my desire to torture people into knowing the *difference* between: 'those who *think* they go with the flow' and those who absolutely '*do* go with the flow' because they are that well trained. And as I said, if the word *script* challenges you, then place the word *template* in its place and you should be just fine. Hmmmm...I feel this house is now clean.

A wee story

Back there on that list you saw me write *pause*. And yes, back in the day a good presenter was trained in the act of knowing when to pause, perhaps to make a point or to build tension. This reminds me of a story told to me by **Gordon Mackie**, a representative of CICA who told me that William Clement Stone's son, **Clem Stone**, had gone out field training with him one day (yep everybody in Mr Stone's organisation had to be able to present in the field, including his own son!). Try as best as you can to imagine this; a corner shop in a 1970's working class inner city. (Aberdeen). The kind of shop that would sell everything from small tins of spam to single cigarettes priced at tuppence, which is 2 old pennies which is the equivalent of 1p today! Suddenly a Silver Cloud Rolls Royce pulls up outside and illegally parks on the corner. Two well-dressed men exit the roller. One of them, the driver, is forty something year old multi - billionaire Clem Stone, who is wearing a silver suit almost identical to the Rolls Royce. The other is a young guy just off the training course, wearing a charcoal grey off the peg suit with three corners of hankie sticking out of the jacket pocket, which was quite trendy for businessmen of the day. They enter the shop and the young guy opens up a leather satchel and goes straight into the pitch to sell the septuagenarian lady an accident insurance policy, which will cover her in the very dangerous job she has in the corner shop, *"…. in any way shape or form and for anything, and that includes at home, at work, at play or even while you are in prison' (seriously, the presentation actually pointed that out!)."* As the presentation continues another three people enter the shop but they just stand there watching the proceedings. British people are trained to queue from birth. Suddenly the man in silver places a had gently on the arm of the other with the three corners of hankie and whispers, very loudly in his ear, in an accent very similar to John Wayne's, *"Steady…"* (however he did not say 'Pilgrim'). The young man visibly twitches with embarrassment. Everyone else just feels awkward. Then John Wayne repeats it twice, very slowly, cautiously even, with the total belief that the lady and the three customers can't hear him…..*"Steady….Steady…. and now….CLOSE!!!!!"* ….as he punches the counter! The young man closed by demanding the money and the woman ran and got her purse, probably with pure relief. Later in the *roller* Clem Stone looked at the man and actually said, *"Awesome pausing by the way. Awesome!"* But yes pausing is important, Indeed I was trained to know when closing (asking for the money!) that at that point I should be silent and simply say the salesman's prayer, which is, *"Help me to keep my big fat mouth SHUT!"* as many trainees go on to talk the client OUT of the sale. They simply cannot be quiet!

And you know what? It can be exactly the same in therapy. Sometimes all the wonderful work is done, but the therapist has a desire to… go on…and on… and on… until a question forms in the mind of the patient: "Maybe this isn't working?"

And so, to cut a long story short I became very successful in the financial services industry because I had developed a track to run on which was transferable in that anyone could understand, teaching many people these skills in order to help others, right up until the time some eejit in the UK Government came up with the idea that self-regulation was a great idea. Then I got to witness a whole industry totally collapse. It wasn't fun. Here's a prediction, if any government in any country in the world sets up a self-regulatory body with the belief that that will be the answer in order to police alternative therapies such as hypnotherapy it will create many jobs and indeed salaries and bonuses: for many *arseholes*. But many hypnotherapists and indeed quite possibly hypnotherapy itself will die. It's Capitalism pure and simple. And is not remotely interested in anything other than producing more capital.

CHAPTER 7

Goldilocks

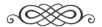

I think it might be a good idea to cover something from way back then that might explain a little bit about how I think today and how I believe it's important that a person in any situation has to be not just trained, but also able to understand *why* they were trained in that particular way, in order that they might, 'pass-on these small but wonderful gifts', which if recognised, will indeed be guaranteed to change the entire world of the recipient. This is also for YOU if you're thinking right now, "I get what Bob is actually saying, but to be honest I'm not sure if I could learn a script, even if it IS a template for success. Hopefully, you will *love* **Goldilocks**.

As I said I spend a great deal of my time sitting across from people informing me that they suffer from extreme anxiety linked to all forms of social settings. This can be anything from asking for a stamp at the post office, going to a function, sitting through a business meeting, making a presentation, telling someone assertively how they feel about a certain situation, going to get a kilt fitted (seriously, these are all from my case studies) or of course that old favourite, public speaking. But we need to fix them. And how do we fix them when we're concerned about *us*? *Our* consultation? How good *we* are? How much *we're* in control!

Welcome to Goldilocks ☺ This is quite possibly my favourite protocol simply because when I got this... I got everything. It awakened me, a sleeping giant! Indeed, it's not so much a protocol but rather a concept. But it is extremely powerful and has carried me through many occasions in my life. And now I pass it on to you. Goldilocks is lovely because it can never fail you and *once you understand and ACCEPT its power,* you will sail through any given situation for the rest of your life with very few problems. I also use this in teaching therapists who, despite having spent thousands of pounds in hypnosis training academies, are still terrified that they might make a mistake in their presentation to either groups or a one on one consultation. THE GOLDILOCKS state of mind stops this from ever happening again. And all they have to do, is let go!

It was back in the 70's and I was in Bradford on a training fortnight for one of the very top direct salesforces worldwide. Our goal was to be able, at the end of the fortnight, to present a ten-minute pitch. That was it. Two weeks away from home, in a hotel, to learn how to deliver a ten-minute pitch. The average demographic in the room would have been mid to late 20's. These people were mainly chosen for their energy. All of their training would be in 'positive mental attitude' and very little else. At the end of the two weeks they would be allowed home... *IF...* they had learned the pitch. If not they would be required to stay there until the trainer was confident they could deliver it effortlessly.

It was my time. I was tense, but I had worked hard for two long weeks.

I remembered many of my friends telling me before I went down to the foreign land that was called England that this was indeed my forte. I was made to be a salesman. "Bobby could sell sand to the Arabs!" one of my best friends would tell everyone. I entered the room and revealed my finely honed skills. And... it was a total nightmare. I was sooooo nervous I simply couldn't concentrate. And the guy behind the desk was a monster of course. Hey, he had to be. That was his role at this time. After 3 or 4 attempts the monster asked me what the problem was. He said he had been taken aback because throughout the fortnight I had been a bit of a star pupil. Of course, I simply told him what he already knew. That I was nervous. I knew that he knew 'the script' and would know every single thing I was supposed to say but not saying properly. He would know the words I was missing out and the other ones I put in which didn't belong there...and... I knew that if I didn't get it right, I wouldn't be allowed home? Rather I'd have to stay over until I learned the pitch perfectly and.... suddenly he held is hand up and threw back his head laughing. And then he stopped becoming a monster and simply said: "Yeah sure we *tell* you that, but we don't really mean it. You're young guys and gals and we don't want you out on the town every night, so we lie to you in order to get you to practice more in the evenings. We tell you that if you can't do the pitch perfectly to us on the second Friday you won't get back to your families. We tell you that we'll keep you here until you learn it. But we know of course that you will already know it. That you'll know it perfectly. But also, we know that you'll have a problem pitching it to *us*, we who can *see* inside your head as you're presenting your talk. But don't worry about that, it's not that important. You're going to be on your train later this afternoon I promise you, because I'm catching the same one!"

I could feel myself seething. Two weeks in a hotel room and now the guy was telling me that it wasn't that important. Then he said, "Look, I want to tell you a story. Sit back in your chair, make yourself comfortable. Okay? So, let me begin......"
And then, I swear, he said: "Once upon a time there were three bears. There was a daddy bear, a mummy, bear and a teensy-weensy baby bear. (*when he said 'teensy weensy baby bear' he made his voice squeak and I wanted to punch him, very much*). Now the three bears lived in a house deep in the woods. But one day they left their home to go into town to buy some groceries. While they were gone a young girl happened to come across their home there in the woods. The girl was very pretty with long blonde hair which hung like gold locks all down her back. In fact, people actually called her, 'Goldilocks' (*and I got even angrier!*). Anyway, she was quite surprised to find this house so deep in the woods and became curious, wondering who lived here. After knocking on the door for some time Goldilocks turned the handle and much to her surprise the door swung open. So, she goes in and steps into the living room where she finds these three chairs. The big one, Daddy Bear's chair is too hard, whilst Mummy Bear's chair, a slightly smaller one, is a little too soft. But Baby Bear's (*squeaky voice again*) chair is just right. Then she decides to enter the kitchen where, much to her surprise she espies three bowls of..... *cornflakes*!" I raised a hand and he stopped talking. "Porridge!" I exclaimed.

"What?"

"Porridge. It wasn't cornflakes. It was three bowls of porridge."

"And how do you know that?" he asked.

"Because I've heard the story before" I almost shouted.

And then the trainer smiled, and simply stated:

"That's right... you daft bastard! *You've* heard the story before. But *they* (he waved his hand to the world outside the window) haven't! They've never heard this story before. They have no idea where you should be pausing, modulating, hesitating, emphasising, or any of the words you should be using or not using. It's not their story Bob. It's *your* story. We know that you know it. And know you can simply go out and tell it anyway you like. You can even make as many mistakes as you want. Intentionally even! They'll always *assume* that you are saying everything 100% accurately, because that is the impression, we have trained you to give them. And that confidence will grow inside you because you have taken a simple script and you have *templated* it!"

(are you *listening* to this reader? Are you *getting* this?)

"You are the only one that knows the story, so you'll know you'll never ever have to worry about getting it right ever again. Because nobody *else* will ever know!"

And...I got it! I understood it perfectly. I simply remember wanting to kiss him! I realised how well I had been trained and knew what I had to concentrate on in order to get to my goals. It's funny because I don't remember the trainer's full name, just that he was called John.

Later when I was promoted and moved to different sales divisions within the company, he did contact me a couple years later to congratulate me on receiving the rewards: *'Sales Representative of the Year'* and we talked about that Friday afternoon. Just a moment. A moment in time when my head went: *boom!*

I tell this story at all my workshops because I find that many people I talk to in these situations are normally anxious in case they foul up. Or rather are anxious about being *seen* to foul up. They're terrified they say the wrong thing, that they screw up on a word or phrase, or even forget where they are in their narrative, talk or presentation. And my message is to stop worrying, and remember that the only way that the person, group or audience KNOW that you've fouled up, is if you convey it to them. Because it's your story. ALL of it. You can't make a mistake even if you *want* to. Go ahead and try, I dare you. If you don't tell your audience that you're screwing up, then they won't know. Because they've never heard *your* story before. And in your story if Goldilocks eats cornflakes then that's the story. 'Goldilocks eats cornflakes'. With this little arrow in one's quiver, there can be no fear of fouling up, making a mistake or being pulled up for getting your story wrong. Because no one KNOWS your story except you. I have treated an army of people over many years suffering from anxiety both in the office and in performance skills such as public speaking, who, once they *truly* grasp and accept the Goldilocks concept, watch those same fears diminish and die. So, we have a Story. An **impregnable template.**

Made impregnable through the skill-set of being able to construct a great script in which we can go for an enjoyable train-ride, enjoying the scenery and making choices where and when we want to exit the train and for how long before stepping back on in order to end a perfect journey and on time.

CHAPTER 8

The Wall (The Initial Consultation)

I think it's now time to look at: The Consultation... through **The Wall.**

When I was asked by Windsor Life Assurance Company Ltd in the 80's to come up with a plan whereby it could be proven that merely by using a set sequence of words the statistics for making appointments could be demonstrably seen by its training department (NLP had just kicked off around this time but it wasn't yet talked about in sales) we agreed that the worst parts of the job when it came to making appointments were in the roles of *telephone* and *cold-canvassing at the door.* A cold call is an unsolicited telephone call, visit or other communication, usually on the part of a business seeking to attract new customers. Here in the UK it died away in the 80's although it is still legal today.

Back in the 70's and early 80's one of the phrases used by sales reps was that the contact with the public was rather like there was this wall between both parties, blocking the representative from 'telling their story'.

In cold canvassing at the door the householder opens the door and sees a business suit and a briefcase and in their minds they immediately build a wall!

In watching the reps cold canvassing I would hear their favourite lines, "Hello there, what a lovely day, I was just wondering if... Hiya, We're just doing a survey... and ...Good afternoon, might I ask you a few questions with regards to…"

It wasn't just the openings and the lines that were poor, but the actual reps themselves had fear in their eyes which was palpable. They looked like *matter out of place*, thus the *feel* was wrong. So, when I went out with a rep we would already talk about this *WALL* and they would always agree that yes, this was indeed the case. So, I told them this:

"We're about to drive to (it would be a rough area of that town). Here's a piece of paper that I want you to read and memorise. When we leave the car, I'm going to knock on doors and I'm going to say what's on the paper which I have already memorised. Your job is to do absolutely nothing. You are going to watch me and hear me say these exact words, which I am using for a reason. When I make 3 appointments we are going to stop. That might be in 10 minutes or several hours. But we won't be stopping until that happens. Have you got all of that?"

"Yes" they would reply.

"And what's your job?"

"To do nothing."

Understand these people were already very highly motivationally trained and in an almost hypnotic setting they had been totally programmed to accept that: *'winners never quit and quitters never win'*. All I had to do was prove that to be the case. To reveal that truth to them. The piece of paper I gave them simply said, *'Hi there, my name is Bob Burns, this is my colleague John Smith, and we are the local representatives for Windsor Life, the insurance and investment people. We're in the area today seeing yourself and all your neighbours mainly to make appointments, to call back at a later date, just to see if we can give any help or advice sometime in the future perhaps. Now we are going to be working here today, this evening and most of tomorrow, when would be the best time for you?'*

Please be aware that I understand completely if you think that's rubbish or it wouldn't work or you'd slam the door in our faces. We get that. That's exactly what *most* householders thought, felt and did! But do understand that all of that was expected and factored in on our part as professional prospectors at that time. We were bell-curving. We simply wanted to see if we had created a difference. And we had. Our success rates much to our surprise were well over 40% higher in making appointments. Let's have a look at why shall we?

Remember we said that true communication really is based upon: *what's said, what's heard, what's understood and what appropriate action is taken.*

Let's have a look at what communication we believe happened (when I say *we* I want to pay tribute to a trainer by the name of Mike Bateson who was a former colonel and a psychologist in the British Army whom I worked with and learned a great deal from).

When the door opened, we would step back and smile, hoping this would nudge the wall down a bit?)

'Hi there, my name is Bob Burns, this is my colleague John Smith and we are the local representatives for Windsor Life, the insurance and investment people. (okay, so mentioning we were local we felt actually helped, however we didn't kid ourselves, we had allowed for the fact that seeing our attire and hearing

94

what we represented the wall would go racing up again!)

We're in the area today seeing yourself and all your neighbours (in the area today, seeing ALL of us)

mainly to make appointments, (they're only making appointments)

to call back (ahh their calling back)

at a later date, (it's going to be later)

just to see (it's only to see)

if we can give (they want to give)

any help (their helping)

or advice (they're just advising)

sometime (It's not now)

in the future (definitely not right now)

perhaps (and it's only perhaps).

Now we are going to be working here today, this evening and most of tomorrow, when would be a good time for you?'

Please understand that while you might be looking at our assumptions and thinking 'that ain't gonna' work we were indeed wondering the same thing. But work they did, the walls came down. We were using scripted argument instead of going with the flow and the difference was *immediately* potent.

I'll say it again. I truly believe that a great therapist is a great salesperson. You get the person, or the part within the person, to buy into YOUR reality and… you have a sale. Your reality becomes their reality. Albeit in therapy the product will be a *feeling* or a *new belief*. What you say they can see they can see, what you say they can feel they can feel and what you say they can do they can do.

In the therapy room **The Wall** is a complete set of protocols and procedures in how to conduct an **Initial Consultation** and not a teaching of any particular method. However, it is my preferred *go to* method. It is now accepted that many times when a client enters a therapy room there is indeed a *kind of* wall between them and the therapist (and very often felt by both) which needs to be removed in order for therapy to take place. When something *doesn't* work experienced therapists do something else, based on their experience and skills. The method that gets used and fixes everyone has not yet been created. However, **The Wall** will indeed be guaranteed to get you that experience and skills and how to develop them in order to turn you into a much better therapist. It's like a standard operational procedure.

STANDARD OPERATIONAL PROCEDURES (SOP)

Every commercial pilot in the world carries a book of 'Standard Operational Procedures' (SOP) Spanish, French and American pilots might all be in the cockpit together but each one (in their own language) will carry their own SOPS. And they will be identical, in order to ensure the plane takes off, flies and lands perfectly, in the right place and at the right time.

(You might even call it a kinda'….. script or a template?)

This why I wanted to devise 'The Perfect Consultation' in order to break down any potential wall which can often stand between the therapist and the client, and keep that train on the rails in order to arrive on time at the end of the session with all the necessary information gathered.

BUT WAIT!!!.....TIME OUT!!! You guys need to know what's going on in the minds of those people who get an appointment with Bob Burns. About 80% of my clients nowadays are personal recommendations. That is rather than someone being simply given my name (a referral) most of my clients are personally recommended to me by someone whom I have worked with already and been able to help. So, I have to confess that that is a huge thing to have in my favour before they even arrive. But you will need to know that I tell them all the same thing on their phone call:

"So firstly I want you to come for an Initial Consultation. This will let me know what I need to know about how you work and whether or not I can hypnotise you or feel that I can work with you. If not I give you your money back (I have never given a client their money back). Assuming all of that is okay we can set up a couple of sessions. Does that sound alright with you?"

Again that is a totally scripted response to an enquiry. I can say that I have never had someone *not* come in for a consultation (or not turn up for one online) on hearing the above. Neither have I ever had anyone *not* come back for sessions after the initial consultation. The exceptions to that rule will be someone perhaps with fear of flying and needing to get on a flight that week and perhaps I genuinely never *need* to see them again. Anyway, let me take you into my bijou therapy room where sometimes magic takes place. **The Consultation** is where the therapist meets the potential client for the very first time. In most situations the therapist will talk over the problem with the client, getting a case history.

Finding out *their* thoughts. Then attempt to ascertain where they (the client) *think* the problem started (they will almost certainly be wrong of course but their thoughts and beliefs may be found to be relevant). Some clients will give a great picture on the reality of their illness, whilst it has to be remembered that with many people their illness is absolutely *their* illness and because it is *their* illness they have complete ownership which gives them the right to *'tell their story'*, seemingly totally unaware that you, the therapist, have had a fair idea of their story from the moment they uttered their first sentence. This is what you do. These are the people you see. Yes we *do* treat the patient and not the illness, however having experienced certain illnesses and phobias so many times the therapists has a strong knowledge of the back story and the effect it will be having on the client as many of the paths of certain illnesses will indeed be very similar.

Of course, we will continually be looking for signs, cracks, traces, hints, differences... and yet they (the client) must never be interrupted during this very important part of the consultation. They will then go on to mention treatment they've already had and if they are undergoing any form of either allopathic medicines or other treatments at this point in time.

Remember that The Consultation is all about welcoming the client and finding out whether or not we can work with them with perhaps a soupcon of hypnosis thrown in. I say a soupcon because sometimes, being a hypnotist in a therapy room we have a tendency to 'be doing hypnosis' even when we are not! Trust me, all hypnotists will *get* that.

It is a way of life for many of us. A good hypnotherapist is a good salesperson and normally a good salesperson is like a good chef. And we become better chefs than most by knowing HOW and WHEN to *sprinkle* and HOW MUCH. 😊 There is a wonderful line from **Don Marquis** (early 20th century humourist and journalist) who opened up my therapeutic mind when I read his words, "An idea is not responsible for the people who believe it." In other words, the hypnotherapist *sells* the idea to the subconscious, which doesn't really know the difference between imagination and reality. *But* the subconscious is a *genius*. It doesn't *need* to know the difference between imagination and reality. It simply knows that if it can get the conscious to believe it (and it always can) then that *becomes* the reality of the client, simply because, **'Reality is Plastic' (Anthony Jacquin).** (Buy this please, you'll love it 😊)

And nothing is more fascinating than to watch someone's life change in what I already said I like to call, 'An *Aha* Moment'. And that often happens when you, the therapist, based on your activity knowledge and know-how and skills, deliver to them a life changing idea in a sentence that touches them in a way that makes their eyes light up like a naked Archimedes having the scientific principles of density and buoyancy slap him in the face, as he masturbates in a bath of rose-petaled water *(your ADD is kicking in Bob. you just wrote that for a bit of fun. Go get yourself a wee Glenmorangie and remember to take that bit out before the book goes to print!).* All therapists know that for something to be achieved it has first to be conceived and then believed. And when that happens... job done! However, we have to first of all acknowledge our client, comfort them, explain to them, reassure them in a way that they can fully understand (or as close as possible) what is about to take place. Remember many clients at this stage are very nervous and they have the three questions that never get vocalised, Who is this? Can I trust them? Should I do what they say? And we of course give the three answers (indirectly) This is who I am. You can absolutely trust me. I just need you to do what I say. And 'Voila'... we're dancing! We just need to know what we need to be working on and when. Sometimes it's the work and sometimes it's the client. Allow me to explain from the mouth of another mentor of mine, One of the greatest card magicians of all time, Madrid's **Juan Tamariz**, who famously said, _"Sometimes in order to do great magic I manipulate the spectators more than the cards."_ ... and I remember thinking, "Yes! Yes of course!" without even contemplating all those years ago that that would become a part of my actual therapy! ☺

And so this is **THE WALL,** A formula which I claim, indeed guarantee, can get any therapist through any initial session, giving them a complete track to run on revealing to the client that they have chosen well. That _this_ is the therapist who can indeed help them. If I had a son, daughter or best friend coming into this business and wanted to have a great opening consultation, THIS is what I would teach them. Here are the 16 parts that make The Wall which I do with every person who enters my therapy room for their Initial Consultation,

Lets have a look at those 16 parts of The Consultation:

1) CHAT (WHY they are here)

2) THE SWAN

3) IMAGINATION

4) CHEVREUL'S PENDULUUM

5) THE WALTZ

6) THE 3 ELEMENTS

7) RESPONSE TESTS (also known by *other* therapists as suggestability tests)

8) HYPNOTISE

9) RELAX

10) RELEASE

11) ADDRESS THE PROBLEM

12) INSERT IMPREGNABLE BUBBLE

13) BLOWAWAY TECHNIQUE

14) CONFIRMATION (if possible)

15) EXPLAIN SESSIONS (book now or check diary)

16) NOTES (including hypnotic rating)

PART 1/16

CHAT

Why they are here to see me is fairly straightforward. They mentioned that at the time of making the appointment. I know that many therapists at this point in time do a full fact find and that's great. Very professional I'd say. But it's not for me. Not yet. Right now, I only want to know if I can work with them. But for now, as I said earlier *they* get to tell *their* story, as I scribble down notes of both what they say and things I maybe notice. Not of their story itself, but in those aha moments, a trace of emotion, a cusp of an abreaction, a sigh, a rub of a forehead, a twitching finger. And next to these things I'll right KI, which means 'key idea' and what I think that spontaneous thought I had at that moment was all about, to be checked at a later time perhaps. The really important thing to remember in the opening chat is that the obvious may only seem obvious or be presented as obvious. It may be that they have recognised something, but falsely, and in doing that they themselves will have constructed *false premises* which in some cases will have thrown they themselves off in all sorts of tangents. Anyway, this is *their* story and it will be highly important for them to be allowed to tell it.

An example might be, *"All of this came about because of how my father mentally abused me after he had retired from 35 years as a postman in Didsbury during which he had an affair with….etc"* And before you know it they're off! Story after story revealing how they are aware of absolutely *everything* including the *cause* of their problem. They know everything linked to the story but can't stop the problem. And have never for a second considered that *that* might not *be* the cause. But as I said whether they do or whether they don't, whether they're right or whether they're wrong. It is their story and they get to own it, change it and tell it. It doesn't matter that they have already told their story to their doctor, consultant psychologist, psychiatrist, cognitive behavioural therapist, a medium, a shaman, each member of their family and all of their friends…continuously, over several years.

They haven't told *you* yet. Let's take a moment. I do hope you find this as interesting as I did; I have worked for many years in the corporate sector mainly being employed to present magical or mind-reading ice breakers or merely to entertain the clients of *my* clients. One day I had a person select a card then put it back into the pack. I then waved my hand over the pack and his card was gone. I then extracted it from the handkerchief pocket of his jacket, which he was wearing as he stood there, three feet from me (a very standard magician's trick). Years later I was in this gentleman's company again where he told the story to the group of what I had done all those years ago. The interesting thing was that in the story *he* told, after the card disappeared it reappeared inside his wallet, which was inside his jacket, which was hanging over a chair 20 feet away. Then he looked at me and smiled as everyone looked at me with amazement. I of course accepted the story as being completely true. But there you go, something all magicians know. That when you perform a miracle for someone it becomes theirs. *Their story.* And they get to do whatever they wish to change that story because it's theirs. Even embellishing it, without even knowing their doing it! There will be millions of people out there whose lives are a mess and yet cannot talk to others about it. They feel they don't understand, but yet we are happy to talk to them about them. And they listen to us as now and again, even in this very early stage of the consultation we can pace and lead our client as we lay the foundations of our *changework*.

Someone once wrote, *"If you talk to a man about himself, he'll listen to you for a thousand years!"* So, when we do talk we talk about *them*, although mainly letting them do most of the talking. As I wrote earlier, we can pace and lead. That is, we can pull them away from certain places in the story and get them to talk about other parts. This is because *right now* they are too close to the mountain to be able to *see* it for themselves.

But we are at a distance and can see it a little clearer, and, like good experienced Sherpas, have climbed this mountain before with many other clients, whom we helped insert their flag when they reached the top. We just cannot tell them that yet. They've told their story already to all the experts and friends remember? And no-one has been able to help them. So, we decorously insert our crampons and ice pics as we guide them on the climb.

So apart from getting their name and contact details in The Consultation, I mainly have at this point in time (again we'll get to all the stuff later, right now I only really need to know if I can work with them) only one question, "Why are you here to see me *today*?" *Today* being the operative word. They could have come last week, month or year but I want to know why *today*. Chances are something has happened and in the asking of that seemingly very simple question they will always find an answer. Even if they did not have one before they arrived! I also want to know *exactly* what the problem is and if they simply say that they just want to be happy I will very often lean forward and tickle them under the armpit, and ask if there is anything *else* I can do for them, with a chuckle of course as I don't want them to know about my touching habit just yet (okay so that's a joke-yeah?).

But I need more from them, specifically, and then they do tell me what their problem is and go on to tell me their story, the one they have told over and over again, because it's important to them to *tell* it. And at the end of their story I will look them straight in the eye and say, *"I don't suppose you brought your manual with you, did you?"* They look quizzical. *"You know, your manual, the book that tells me exactly how you work, so if you had say a fear of spiders I'd simply look up, o,p,q,r,s...sp, spi, spiders. And it would tell me exactly what to do to fix you... yeah?"*

They will at least smile at this point and say "NO". I then go on: *"Okay, so here's the good news! You don't have an actual problem."* They look at me puzzled. *"By that I mean you don't have a conscious problem, because if it were a conscious problem, you'd know what that was and you would have fixed it yourself by now. You simply wouldn't put up with this. Isn't that true?"*

So, reader this is where you have to stay with me and believe what I'm saying here. And I need you to believe me for two reasons, 1) because it's true and 2) because it will save you a lot of time in the wilderness. Okay? 😊

They *always* answer YES to this question. ALWAYS! They *get* it! Then I continue... *"So that tells me that you have a SUBconscious problem. And that tells me that it's all actually INside you, and yet, it's totally OUTside your control. Does that sound about right?"* And again, they will *always* answer YES to this question. ALWAYS! *"That's why it's so difficult to shift. And that means that I have to ignore you consciously, no matter what you think or feel it is, and go talk to your subconscious, or a part within your subconscious. Does that make sense?"*

I think this is a nice mellifluous statement. It can be highly pleasing to the ear of the anxious soul sitting before me. Indeed, at this point 99% of people will nod their head in agreement and even give me a smile. It's the first *eureka moment* of the therapy for them (I *love* eureka moments and try to fill my therapy room with them) which I strongly feel lifts a weight from the shoulders of this stranger who is about to become my client ... *(a client is someone who sees me in two or more sessions, as opposed to a one session customer, which I find distasteful).* So here we are. We take around 30 seconds (yes I *have* timed it) to ask and get *three* YES answers which completely relaxes the client and gives them *four* new facts:

1) they don't have a conscious problem
2) they have a subconscious problem
3) it's all inside of them...
4) ... and yet it's totally outside of their control

My next statement is, *"Great, so I don't want you to fight me but neither do I want you to help me, I simply want you to allow me to do my work. Is that okay?"* And boom... another YES. I then close with: *"So, your job is to do nothing. What's your job?"* I simply love affirmative questions. And they reply: *"To do nothing."*

(just like all those trainee salespeople standing next to me, trembling slightly as I showed them how to cold-canvass a whole street all those years ago)

And now they can relax and let me begin to do my work.

It's then I throw the client off their feet by simply asking, *"Are you left-handed or right-handed?"* ....and it's round about then that somehow, I *always* begin to hear wings flapping as The Swan gets ready to land... LOL!!!

PART 2/16 THE SWAN

Which we talked of earlier. But I want to clearly state that I was already a very successful therapist doing only this form of consultation long before I discovered and constructed The Swan, The Wall holds good on its own...I promise!

PART 3/16 IMAGINATION

As I finish The Swan Protocol I immediately ask, *"Tell me, do you think you have a good imagination?"* I simply want to know if they are visual. So, after I get them to close their eyes, I ask... *"In your imagination, can you see a white horse?"* I do not *just* ask them, *"CAN you see a white horse?* But rather I add *"IN your imagination"* Remember Communication being what is, said... heard... understood... what action is taken. It is entirely possible for someone who can see a white horse IN their imagination to answer you 'NO' if you don't make clear you mean *in* their imagination. Remember that little things are important.

Bill Duncan was my main mentor in the world of magic and went on to become one of my very best friends. I truly believe he was one of the sharpest of any human beings I have ever met and definitely one of *the* loveliest. Today Bill has Alzheimer's and no longer performs. Indeed, he no longer recognises me.

But he has given me a wealth of knowledge and ideas over many years, some of these without even trying. *The Imaginary White Horse* was one of those, but purely by accident!

My wife Leigh and I were visiting one evening and Bill had cooked us a meal. We were talking about imagination and I said, "It's kinda' like, well, close your eyes for a sec. Now then Bill if I asked if you could see a white horse you can do that very easily, yeah? But you know it's not actually there. Now then..." At this point Bill interrupted me and said, "Yes but I can't actually *see* a white horse" And I replied, "No of course you can't. But you *can* see it in your *imagination*, yes?" and Bill replied, "I don't know what you mean." Remember, this is one of the sharpest people that I have ever known. I was stunned. I had assumed that this is how *we* work. That *all* of us have this ability to tap into our imagination and create almost any *other* reality. As the conversation went on Leigh and I discovered that Bill was *different* to us (Leigh and I). That is to say he had no *visual* imagination. And to us, both social scientists with pretty decent maps of the world, we were amazed. So was Bill.

This of course is called *Aphantasia*, a word first coined by Sir Frances Galton (an incredible polymath) way back in 1880. And it simply means that a person cannot create imagery in their mind's eye. For what it's worth I have learned over the years that this type of person, when asked to imagine, say, a white horse, will often do it by simply hearing their own voice in their head repeating over and over *"white horse, white horse, white horse"*. We then discovered lots of other skills that Leigh and I, through pure coincidence both had.

I should very quickly add that in reality it's not really a skill. Although there is a claim from a certain Dr Zeman that it is hereditary or environmental, my experiences would suggest that that is *not* completely true since my own work has had me getting involved with many families who differ hugely. Although this form of imagination (visualisation) can indeed be taught, practiced, and learned. It can even be honed and sharpened. However, in my experience, for many it doesn't happen quickly. And remember visualisation isn't really vision per say, although to people like me it can be even *stronger than the real thing*, seriously. But through investigating with lots of subjects we get to gain experience and develop an *activity knowledge* of how this form of imagination can be... *tweaked*. For example, if they have a grandchild and they love that grandchild, and I suddenly ask them to stop thinking of the horse (which they couldn't see) any more, but to now imagine seeing their grandchild, in their imagination, perhaps 'picking wild flowers for them then turning and smiling as they hand them over', very often they start giggling as this kicks in, and in many cases it can happen immediately! Now I know that non visualisers find it difficult to believe that members of their family have this skill (and vice versa of course). That this family has been together for all their lives and have never known of these differences. Well, that's because of assumption. It would appear that in this field we all *assume* that we are the same. For me, if I could not *see* inside my mind every second of every moment (and I *do*) I think I might very well go mad! But if I had never developed this ability, I would most probably never think about it.

I guess it might be like this with awareness itself. So, try this. If you haven't done so already, why not close your eyes and find out about yourself right now? I simply want you to close your eyes and see if, *in your imagination*, you can see a white horse. Go ahead, try that right now! Your eyes are now open again aren't they? I knew it! I love being *psychic!!!* Well? Did you see the horse? And I know that for some of you it turned into a unicorn! We'll talk about that when we meet 😊

After asking my client whether or not they can see a white horse I go on to ask them to close their eyes, think of a piece of music or song that they love, and to nod to me when they have thought of a piece. It's strange but I promise that you will find that many people 'in the moment' simply cannot think of *any* piece of music. Do not let this go on for too long as it breaks the pace. If they haven't got anything by ten seconds, I ask them to think of the song: 'Happy birthday to you'. Then the same again, I ask them to imagine they can hear the music.

I follow this by asking them again to close their eyes, then imagine that I am walking behind them and then placing my hands onto their shoulders..... *"Now"*. Just for the hell of it I follow this up by asking them to imagine smelling a bunch of flowers and tasting, whether they like curry or not, a spoon full of curry. So... for those who see the white horse I immediately scribble into their notes that they have some form of *clairvoyance*. Now look I don't wish to have you guys running back and forward into the internet to check out the real origins and meanings of words. Suffice to say that clairvoyance originates from French: clair = clear and voyance = vision.

Thus, a clairvoyant is simply one who sees clearly. And yeh yeh yeh I know some of you will be saying, "Ah but it's linked to extrasensory perception" but guess what? To those that do *not* have the gift it bloody well *is* extrasensory perception! All of it!

And so we have:
clairvoyance......... clear seeing
clairaudience........ clear hearing
clairsentience.......clear feeling
olfactory...............smelling
gustatorial.............tasting

The American hypnotist Anthony Galie often talks about the best subjects being excellent visualisers and I would agree with that. Indeed, for hypnotic procedures it might be argued that we would prefer them to possess the ability to imagine in the fields of sight and hearing and feeling. But none are really necessary. Indeed, they will begin to pick up on these latent gifts *in* hypnosis. However, by asking these questions I am now learning to know my client. At the end of this section on imagination I will often say, *"So, remember when you walked in here? I said I wasn't too sure how to treat you because you never brought your manual and I don't know you or know anything about how you work? Well, guess what? I know much more about you now."*

And I do know more about them if I wish to use it. If I want to ask them a positive question and they couldn't have seen a horse there is very little point in me saying, "Do you see what I'm saying?"

Because even if they understand me, they might just *say* "no" because they actually don't *see* what I'm saying. But if I they felt my hands on their shoulders and I say, "Can you feel where I am on this?" they may smile and tell me that yes, they do indeed *feel* what I'm saying. It *feels* right to them. This is *them*. This is *their* manual we are developing. This is what *they* do and how *they* work. And now, (not based on the NLP course I went on and took notes but rather what they *told me about themself* two minutes ago) I have information. The map is *becoming* the terrain! And it's a map that we can use to communicate later. Remember (once more) what we said about communication. It's what is, said, heard, understood and the action taken (yeah I know I've already said that 6 times. Ther'll be more, trust me!)

PART 4/16 CHEVREUL'S PENDULUM

Remember, no one says we can't have fun in the therapy room. And the fascinating work of this 19th century French chemist is something I use at this point in the session for two reasons. First of all it is simply such a wonderful thing to do in that it puts a little bit of fun into the therapy, but more importantly it delivers a truly beautiful explanation of how we (a part *within* their subconscious and me) are going to *maybe* fix them (see **time out** in next paragraph). And they get to understand all of that inside 60 seconds! It's a wonderful phenomenon and every time I hear a therapist say, *"yeah it's okay but y'know I don't use the pendulum myself, as it's all nonsense"* my eyes go glazy and saliva trickles out the side of my mouth and I truly want to stab them in the jugular with my ball point pen (and it's not a cheap one) as I hum, 'Non, Je Ne Regrette Rien' (as a tribute to Chevreul the Swinger). That's how angry these people can make me!

Time Out...

At this present moment in time I am in the middle of doing several online workshops with many people from all over the world.

This past weekend I was working with a very large group and one of the ladies pulled me up on a remark I had made (see last paragraph) and told me she found it challenging that I used and *do* use the word FIX as in 'fixing them' as she pointed out: "People are not broken. We don't need fixing" she informed me.

Now I should add that she was very well mannered and I got totally where she was coming from. But just so that you the reader understand I'm NOT in that camp of where: 'All we really need is more self-love and self-acceptance and an opportunity to grow'. It's all absolutely lovely. However, here it comes: I see many people who are, beyond any shadow of a doubt... *totally* broken . And I try to fix them. And THAT is the language I use when talking to them. The rest is someone else's narrative, but not mine. Okaydokay? 😊

So let's move on.

Now I do know that the pendulum is known the world over by associates of pregnant women. And by accosting these pregnant women and holding them down and swinging the pendulum around their open palm, dependent on how it swings (normally to and fro for a boy and around in a circle for a girl) they can tell them the sex of the child.

And get this... they are *never* wrong. You will never hear of a time when they pulled out their pendulum (that didn't sound right I know) and used it on Mary and told her it would be a boy but it was a girl. That narrative has never taken place. However, what *truly* happens is that they are correct 50% of the time which they talk about *forever*. The other 50% simply gets *genuinely* forgotten.

However, in the therapy room, the pendulum has a far better use. For me I like to simply pick it up and say, *"Have you seen this?"* I tell them that as the pendulum hangs there motionless I am about to imagine that there on the carpet is a line going from left to right, and that is all I am now concentrating on. And of course, they see how the pendulum begins to move to and fro. Then I tell them I am now thinking that that line is inside a circle there on the carpet and I am now concentrating on that circle going round and round and... as I speak the pendulum begins to spin around and around. Sometimes I'll go back to the straight line again but when I want to I simply stop, look at them and utter the words: *"Now in all fairness I could well understand if you think I'm cheating so, here, why don't you try it?"*
And I hand them the pendulum, show them how to hold it (best is between thumb, forefinger, and middle finger) and suggest they put their elbow on their knee to support it. I then ask them to gaze at the carpet and off we go. I can say that this works more than 95% of the time! I can also say that when it does not you can actually see them fighting it, which in itself is I feel quite fascinating. Although this can be used in many magical effects, I always tell the client immediately that it has nothing to do with

magic or indeed hypnosis. But rather it is the work of **Michel Eugene Chevreul** who used the concept of the pendulum (circa mid-19th century) in order to discover (or claim) that information held within the subconscious mind could be revealed! Basically, the minute movement of the subconscious is magnified through a heavy weight hanging from a chain or piece of string. Called **Ideomotion**, we can see fibre, nerve and muscle movement without any actual conscious effort. All we need do is make a suggestion to the client to imagine a line going to and fro or a circle going round and round and within seconds the pendulum will do whatever they are thinking. Indeed, this is so strong that many hypnotherapists have seen this as more of a convincer of hypnosis (to the client) than a test. Although it is believed that its origins were meant to be presented as permissive it can be used as either a permissive or an authoritative test. So, the therapist needs to pay attention in how they conduct **Chevreul's Pendulum**. Although as I said in using an imaginary line in the carpet this is how the test is normally done *or* with the pendulum held in the centre a few inches above a drawing (see below) and then asked to imagine.

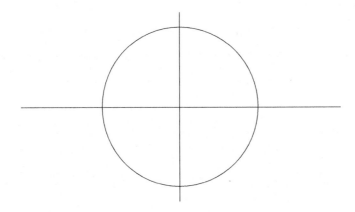

It is to be remembered that if someone cannot do this test then it is possible that the subconscious is fighting it. Some even say that it is the *critical factor (or faculty)* within them that is doing the fighting. But in my findings, I would report that it's more a case of them consciously being concerned or even slightly scared. The fact is that nearly all my clients who fail this test will be in my therapy room asking to be treated for anxiety! However, as therapists it is our job to handle this. I always tell the client my reasons for using the pendulum. It is quite simply to reveal what I feel is a beautiful analogy, for we are sitting together, watching the subconscious buy into an idea. And when the subconscious buys into an idea... *everything* changes. The subconscious does not realise the difference between imagination and reality, but it knows that if it can simply get the conscious (or client) to merely *imagine...* then that *becomes* their reality. Job done! Thus I strongly recommend that if you use Chevreul's Pendulum you follow through with this statement:

"So, if this were a little less than 300 years ago you and I would be burned at the stake for witchcraft!" The client will always laugh along with you…. *"…and yet there is nothing spooky or esoteric about this. Rather its founder, a French chemist called Michel Eugene Chevreul, realised exactly what was happening. Basically, it's you. Or rather that part of you deep within your subconscious, moving all the nerves and fibres of your arm and hand in order to move in the area it desires. And yet it has nothing to do with witchcraft. Indeed, that telling the sex of the child depends on what the person holding the*

116

pendulum THINKS the sex will be, even SUBconsciously, and moves it accordingly! If you like, we might call this psychosomatic. That is that <u>psycho the mind tells soma the body what it thinks</u>, and soma the body acts accordingly, yes?"

They will get this *completely* because they just witnessed it happen in *their* hands!

These next words are very, very, VERY powerful!!!:

"And so we can clearly see, in all forms for example of psychosomatic illness that if psycho the mind can tell soma the body that it's ill, then it's perfectly understandable, through hypnosis, how we can ALSO get psycho the mind to tell soma the body that it's well, yes?"

And voila! The client GETS IT! And don't forget that the subconscious (or a part within the subconscious) is also in the room listening intently. They understand perfectly. And we have now created yet another belief (they're building up YES?). And you are now taking care of problems before they even get to arise! 😊 But hey, let me show you what I mean,

<u>*So get online and look this up:*</u>

CLIP 2 *YouTube:* Chevreul's Pendulum

So, I roll the pendulum up and place it gently in its box. I have always felt that the pendulum should be totally respected. Why? I guess one *could* believe that even if there is no actual magic involved the pendulum itself possesses a certain energy and if so that respect might well be reciprocated. It's a little bit WooWoo maybe, but then again I *am* a little bit WooWoo. Then I congratulate my client on how well they are doing (we call this brush strokes! Remember?)☺

PART 5/16 The Waltz

Then, just as an aside I ask my client, "By the way do you have any idea how people actually get hypnotised?" (a preamble question to The Waltz) This is a very important question as sometimes, if you're very attentive they will relay to you exactly how they would expect to be hypnotised. And every hypnotist totally understands the power of expectancy. But 99% of the time they will say "no" and that is an opportunity for me to say the following:

"It's funny but many people think we simply ask you to 'stare into my eyes' (and I stare into their eyes at the same time) but in the therapy room I don't really do that, or making one's voice go deeper or swinging a watch. But, although I can indeed do all of that, the hypnosis I use in the therapy room is more like teaching someone how to do a Waltz. The thing to remember about teaching anyone how to dance is to remember the student must never, fight the teacher, or try to help them. All the professional dancers from 'Dancing with The Stars' or 'Strictly Come Dancing' will say that all they really want in the early days is for the subject to ALLOW the professional to lead them. Not try to fight them but neither to try to help them. Rather simply ALLOW them to do their work. So for example, if I were wishing to teach you how to do a waltz, I would simply ask you to place your right hand in my left hand and your left hand on my shoulder, as I gently hold you by the waist. Then I would very decorously turn you here and there as we stepped slowly. If anyone came in the room, they'd simply think we were doing a form of a waltz. It might not be a great waltz, but it would get better and better, simply because you're not trying to fight me, you're not trying to help me. You're simply ALLOWING me to do my work. Does that make sense?"

You have now very clearly stated intention of what you are about to do and how you wish them to behave during the procedure. Not fighting you, not trying to help, but simply relaxing and *allowing* you to do your work (And yes, of course it could be argued that you have more than slightly opened the door of further suggestion)

PART 6/16
THE THREE ELEMENTS
a) Conscious
b) Critical Factor (The Viking)
c) Subconscious

There is a phrase in psychology, magic, mentalism and hypnosis, 'Lies to Children'. Basically it suggests that often we will tell a lie to the child (mainly through misrepresentation or omittance) as it suits a particular time in their growth and adjustment to the world, and then at a later date, when they are ready for a more sophisticated truth, we give it to them. In a way this can happen in therapy. For example, we don't really know if there is such a thing as a critical factor, yet the therapist says:

"You will remember that earlier we agreed (WE agreed!) that you don't have a conscious problem, but rather it's a subconscious problem?" Client confirms, ... *"And yet I am talking to you consciously right now. But I really want to go where the problem lies, over there in the subconscious. The challenge is that in order to do that I have to pass that part in the middle that lies between the conscious and the subconscious. And we call this (nodding our head) the **critical factor**."* The client will *always* nod their head also as you say this, even slightly.

The therapist continues, *"And isn't it strange that even right now you're nodding your head whilst thinking to yourself, 'what does he mean, a **critical factor?"*** (they will normally smile or laugh at this point) *That's what it does, the **critical factor**. It critiques every single thing you become aware of. Even while getting you to nod your head to appease me whilst it thinks!"* (again, nearly always the client will smile with the thought of this).

"Indeed, the critical factor *to me is like a seven-foot-tall Viking who is standing before me with his arms folded high on his chest as he says to me, 'You're not getting in!'* (said in a Norse-like voice! ☺)

And it's part of my job to make friends with this Viking, to tickle him perhaps or cajole him in order that he steps aside and lets me in. And the good thing is that the **subconscious** *is begging the Viking to step aside as it wants to play. The* **subconscious** *is kinda' like a seven-year old genius. It doesn't know the difference between imagination or reality but doesn't need to. As we've already seen here today if it can get you to simply imagine something then that* **becomes** *your reality!"*

So what we've done here is to lightly educate our client as to the differences between the conscious and subconscious whilst revealing the relevance of the critical factor (which of course, *real or imagined*, is the model we wish to use at this point in time…to the *child*).

And now it's time to find out a little more about how they work. I personally will often use *this* true story to the client as an explanation or even a small icebreaker for what I'm about to do….

My Canadian Psychologist

So, you may have noticed by now that I like small things. Little differences that can make big differences. minutiae. touches, brush strokes, hints, feints, misdirection, sleights.

I often enjoy telling the client about this young psychologist (true story) who contacted me several years ago from Canada. He was learning the art of hypnosis and he informed me that his 'suggestibility tests' weren't working, and he wanted to know why. I told him that this was most probably because he was an idiot (I said this of course in jest) as he shouldn't be calling them suggestibility tests! Certainly not to the client. People don't want to believe they are thought of as being *merely* suggestible. But rather he should have been using the term: *Response Tests* (obviously you can also use the word, *responsive)*. People simply *love* responsive tests if they are explained properly. And I then explain to my client that we do responsive tests in order to find out possibly where in this wonderful hypnotic ladder they might be, allowing for the fact that they might be slightly nervous that particular day. But alleviating any worries by telling them, *"Don't worry, you'll absolutely love it, I promise!"* So, through **The Swan** (as we shall see) the client can open up and allow that part within the subconscious to reveal itself. We have also ran some small tests to see how their **Imagination** works and both how different and strong these five senses are. Then we touched on how psychosomatic illness can work and how it can begin to be fixed through something as simple as **Chevreul's Pendulum.** We then talked about how we the therapist like to operate within our particular style of hypnosis through the analogy of **The Waltz,** *clearly* stating that we need the client to, not fight us nor try and help us, but simply *allow* us to do our work, before talking about: **The Three Elements** where we brought in the *critical factor,* explaining to the client that they have this kind of *hidden observer* which is always watching over them. We are now getting closer to the moment where we are about to use hypnosis. But first we want to see how the client responds to basic suggestion. How good a subject are they? And it's here where we have the opportunity to introduce and perform *Response Tests* (not suggestion tests, remember? Although they might be? 😊)

PART 7/16   PERFORM RESPONSE TESTS

The response tests come in four areas. They are a) magnetic fingers b) magnetic hands c) light hand and heavy hand d) the hand stick (although yes there are many more)

I don't mind failing whilst working with students, indeed I consider it important for students to both SEE me fail and notice my attitude to failure.

It is also perfectly alright to fail in the therapy room but extremely important not to be *seen* to be failing in anything we *do* in the therapy room. Thus, a lot of thought must go into the framing of these tests. For example, they are not actual tests. Rather we are now approaching this thing called hypnosis and at this point we want to find out a little more about how they the client *works*. So here the therapist might say, *"You remember when you arrived, I noticed that you weren't carrying a manual. So, we now know that you actually don't have one, no? So, since you don't have a manual this is where I REALLY get to know how you work, and I'm going to get a good idea about that simply by completing a short set of what we call, response tests. Although that's actually a misnomer because as I said they're not actually tests. Rather they simply give me some feedback on how you actually work. So, remember The Waltz? All you need to do is simply remember not to fight me but not to try and help me either. You'll actually enjoy this, I promise. All you have to do is ALLOW me to work, okay?"* (notice how the word ALLOW gets used throughout the entire consultation) ... allow...allow...allow...why, you could be excused for thinking I'm using hypnosis! ☺)

We then go through the response tests.

After talking to many hypnotists from the world of street, stage and the therapy room I have never had one disagree with the following:

a) **magnetic fingers** (eyes open) is fantastic, and although even with this alone a person *can* go into hypnosis it is mainly used to see if the subject is going to fight us.

b) **magnetic hands** (eyes closed) is similar and yet it is a sign of how they react to suggestion.

c) **heavy hand light hand.** (eyes closed) The heavy hand is suggestion while it is strongly believed that the hand that rises is indeed an excellent sign of hypnosis beginning to take place. I call this *cusping* because they are indeed cusping on the edge of hypnosis.

d) **hand clasp** (also known as the hand stick) it is mainly accepted that when the hands stick *it is caused by the lactic acid building up in the fingers.* however it can be seen as a convincer thus that in itself has value.

However, YES the client can indeed slip into hypnosis with this or any of the other response tests!

(apologies to experienced hypnotists having to read through this next part)

So, the finger response test is where, with eyes open they clasp their hands together but hold their forefinger together and straight up in the air. The hypnotist asks them to look at their forefingers before saying: "In a minute, but not yet (remember to say 'but not yet' as many people will totally ignore you and open their fingers) I'm going to ask you to open those fingers as wide as you can, then I'm going to snap my fingers and something strange will happen" and then snap your fingers… "and suddenly your forefingers simply want to come together!" The magnetic-hand test is done as the hypnotist asks them to hold their open palms out in front of them and about six inches apart. Then they are instructed to close their eyes:

"… and now I want you to imagine that two pieces of metal are strapped to you palms but as I snap my fingers these two pieces of metal turn into two of the strongest magnets possible, and you can feel those hands being pulled together *now* (snap!), stronger and stronger" etc

And the heavy hand/light hand is where both arms are placed out in front, palms open and the left hand turned upwards whilst the right stays face down.

Here of course they are asked to imagine a heavy bucket being placed on the left hand and gradually filling with water whilst around the wrist of the right hand is tied a piece of string which is attached to a huge red balloon, way up in the air. And whilst the bucket fills with water the balloon has more and more hydrogen air pumped into it making it rise as it tugs and pulls at the right arm, lifting it higher and higher all the way up to the sky.

Indeed, lets show you THOSE FIRST THREE RESPONSE TESTS
1) magnetic fingers 2) magnetic hands 3) heavy/light hands

So get online and look this up:

Clip 3 YouTube: First three response tests)

So after the Heavy/Light Hand test comes The Hand Clasp (by most hypnotists) Personally, I never do a *hand clasp* in the therapy room one-on-one. I would only do that in a stage or group setting. Hey, it's fun! But as I said earlier it is mainly caused by a build up of lactic acid in the fingers and at this stage I want to be more sure. Rather I do a loose hand by their side and the other stuck to the table or chair. For me this matches the light hand performed earlier with regard to eliciting hypnosis. However, for me I make it sound totally unimportant for it to actually work, rather I say:

"I simply want to know at the end of this if you notice any difference whatsoever between the right hand and the left hand. Is that okay? So, don't worry, I don't expect anything to happen."

ONE MORE TIME:

1) "I simply want to know at the end of this if you notice any difference whatsoever between the right hand and the left hand"

2) "I DON'T expect anything to happen!!!!" Then if the sticking *doesn't* take place I simply ask if they noticed any difference between the two hands as I *only* said it might, thus, **no failure has taken place no matter what happens** BECAUSE I clearly said that I only wanted to see if they noticed any *difference*. Even if no phenomena takes place, they nearly always say they did indeed at least feel a difference. I answer by telling them, *"Fine, excellent, that's all I need to know, thank you."* But let's SEE how all of that works eh?

Clip4...*YouTube:* Successful handstick

Clip5 ...*YouTube:* Unsuccessful handstick......
SPOT THE DIFFERENCE!!!

So, as you can see. When things fail, I simply don't mention it. Remember I simply informed them that I wanted to know if they noticed any difference between the right hand and the left hand. And… they did! However, I added many professorial touches (flick of glasses, hand through hair, sniff and stroking of goatee beard. If you are a woman and do not have a goatee beard you simply adjust your bra strap). and I looked busy by writing my notes… although when something does NOT work, I don't actually write anything down. Remember??? Rather I merely pretend to. I just scribble…kinda' like mini mountains? Which in my personal notes simply means: 'It didn't work Bob!' ☹

Remember, I feel that it's important that although I experience many failures in my therapy room, I am never *seen* to fail by the patient. And yes of course in reality there is no failure or success. Rather we get to witness how all these very different people actually work. That's all that is really happening. But remember the saying, 'Lies to Children? In my home I actually have framed above the fireplace in Latin, the 'Burns Family Motto', which is: **'Snekarios Estas Bestas'** which simply means, **'Sneaky Is Best'**…

And I simply would not lie about a thing like that. ☺

But again, all of the above is only there in order for me to know how my client works just that little bit more. I am totally aware that many therapists do no hypnotic testing whatsoever during hypnotherapy. I think it best if I were to simply say I have no idea why they do not and simply leave it at that. Suffice to say that many years ago I trained as a hypnoanalyst where it wasn't required to seek any evidence whatsoever as to whether or not the client (or the hypnotist!) had any hypnotic skills. Looking back this was and is very much a bad idea. *Check* your work. *Know* your client!.

Anyway, now our client is ready to be hypnotised. Truth be known there is a strong chance they have already popped in and out of hypnosis a couple times by now!

But now it's time. There is a saying in the world of magic, *'The amateur magician knows a thousand tricks, while the professional magician knows seven'* and so it should be with hypnosis. Off the top of my head I can think of 37 inductions. Now in the early days I was taught to find the correct induction to fit the subject. However, my experience eventually told me to learn ONE induction really, really well, and then **get all the subjects to fit *that* induction.** In my therapy room I use hand to head induction which works every time. Or at least efficiently enough for what I am now about to do. Remember you have already put in place loads of hypnotic work. They are indeed ready to *run* into hypnosis by this time.

I mentioned Anthony Galie earlier on. When I was talking to him recently in a skype chat he made me giggle as he said very matter of factly, *"If they GO into hypnosis you simply place them into hypnosis, and of course you can use anything. If they don't GO into hypnosis you won't be able to put them into hypnosis."* And of course, he's correct. He made me giggle again when I put it to him that most skilled hypnotists in the world would agree that the percentage of somnambulists who fall into hypnosis (for the quality needed for stage hypnosis say) was 5%,

Meaning 1 in 20 would be a great subject and if you had a room of 100 then you would be fairly confident in having 5 good subjects. But as I said 5% Anthony retorted like lightening, *"Actually it's 2.18% Bob."* I could see he wasn't smiling and said it really confidently, and he went on to tell me that he had put in many years finding that out. Like I said he looked serious, but he was maybe taking the piss out of me LOL!!!

I don't know. He's Anthony Galie for Chrissakes! It was a complete pleasure talking to him ☺.

Anyway, let's get to it shall we…?

PART 8/16 HYPNOTISE

Just as an aside I have this kind of thing I like to do, where just before I do the actual hypnosis I like to ask the client, *"So just as a matter on interest, if I had a magic wand and I could wave it in the air in order for you to know that something had happened today, that you would know a change had taken place, what would that be?"* And I write down exactly what they tell me (something we'll cover later). As I said I normally use only one induction in the therapy room during my Initial Consultation. Any sessions afterwards I can simply tell them to close their eyes and go into hypnosis. That is all that's required. But that induction I do is a hand to head induction, which I believe is one of the favourites of most hypnotists. Remember, that's for a reason yeah? So, I go to shake their hand lift it above their head and tell them to look at their hand as I lift it above their head, pick a spot on it and listen to my voice. After a moment, the hand will feel like it's being drawn to their forehead (because I tell them so), their eyes will become heavy. They can then close their eyes and allow the hand to gently fall down to their side as they allow themselves to go deeper and deeper as they simply drift and dream and tune into the timbre of my voice. Just the vibration of my voice as….etc.

But…! The world has changed has it not? And all my work for over a whole year now has been done 'on-line'! Here it comes again folks: *"Every adversity brings with it the seed of an equivalent or greater benefit"*, … and much to the surprise of myself and many of my colleagues we have been able to discover that certain methods which we would never before have attempted actually work perfectly well. We find for example that an on-line induction works (providing you have of course already put in the work we have already covered during the session) simply by telling them to close their eyes!

So listen up here. All the experienced hypnotists and therapists will watch this and smile knowing that this simply works, okay? All the work needed has been already inserted. On an online induction in a therapy session this is all that is *ever* needed. So remember the KISS principle: *Keep It Simple Stupid:*

Clip 6) *YouTube:* **INDUCTION CLIP**

The other induction I will sometimes use is if I have acquired the knowledge during our discussion that they are somnambulistic and to save time I will simply do a hand-drop. The hand-drop is where I ask them to place their open hand on my open hand, look into my eyes and press as hard as they can, and simply give the command SLEEP as I pull my hand away and catch them incase they slip to the side.

I might add however that on doing sessions *online* I get exactly the same result by simply telling them to look up at a spot on the wall or ceiling and: *"simply tune into the timbre of my voice, just the vibration of my voice, and as your eyes feel heavier you simply…"* etc.

For me it works identically.

Deepeners?

Now I don't wish to go off on a tangent here arguing about whether or not deepeners are needed once a person is IN trance. Old School says yes whilst New School *seems* to say no. Why, there are even arguments as to whether or not there is such a thing as TRANCE!

Yes I do indeed find myself saying: *"and you can now simply allow yourself to go deeper and deeper all the way down"* although very often it is simply not needed. However let's take a moment and talk about hypnotists and hypnotherapists and the differences in the style of their training. I don't believe anyone would argue with me if I were to say that most hypnotherapists would have been trained in slow deepeners whilst pure hypnotists would have been trained to deepen much faster (unless of course it is a theatrical deepener to a crowd on stage (which can be all part of the show). I also believe it would be fair to say that arguably the most popular deepener most use might be the *arm-drop* (not to be confused with the closely named *hand-drop* which is used not for a deepener but rather for a quick induction as explained above).

The arm-drop deepener is where, immediately after induction, the hypnotist lifts the arm of the sitter by the wrist and gives it a little shake before telling them that: *"…and when I drop your arm down to your lap you will allow yourself to go even deeper, all the way down to a profound sense of…"* etc

If I'm being honest I have used this for years. If I'm being *more* honest it's simply because my findings clearly indicate by their body language that *they* believe they are going deeper. I have no idea why many 'new kids on the block' have a burning desire to change standard hypnotic belief. For example they say that there is no such thing as trance *(and in a voice that states they know this for a fact which really pisses me off but they don't know that cause I'm nice and just smile quietly)* whilst the person is sitting there with their eyes rolled back and saliva gushing from their mouth. And there's a reason for that…it's called 'being in trance'!

Anyway, while we're here I want to take the trouble to share with you a wee protocol I constructed a few years ago, but purely by accident. I strongly urge you to try it, you'll like it! ☺. I give you:

The Cascade

It came about in the middle of me doing an arm drop (in order to deepen the trance state, *assuming there is such a thing*) with this client, and as I dropped their arm a little too early. When I did this I tried to catch their hand but I missed it *again*. And blow me if I didn't miss it the *third* time before it landed on their thigh.

BUT... as I looked at them their head was nearly hitting their belly button. So I woke them up... cleared them... and did the whole thing again (remember Goldilocks?).

I induced them... but then I *told* them what was about to happen:

"AS I drop this hand you'll feel it hit my hands a couple times on the way down. And with each hit you will allow yourself to go deeper and deeper, all the way down."

Then much to my surprise I watched them go down and down and down and down into a seemingly profound state. It was kinda' like a four for one? 😊 And I should say that later I started to make a sound like *boom* with my mouth with every connection of their lowering hand hitting mine? Starting high and going lower with each hit. It reminded me of the score music for the famous British soap: *Eastenders.* And for what it's worth I feel that because I *pantomime* this... it actually helps. As I often say: 'Nobody says you can't have *fun* in the therapy room!'

Let me show you here:

Clip 7)...*YouTube:* THE CASCADE

PART 9/16 RELAXATION

The next thing of course is simply to relax them, as we say, 'all the way down'. We have already looked at the arguments that in hypnosis they don't need to be deepened, or even in a trance. I'd go even further and say that they don't even need to be in hypnosis (**The Swan** clearly reveals that to us)! However, I don't want to have any more arguments with a 14-year-old expert who has seen stuff on Youtube and now wants to have a philosophical argument with me online. Hypnosis is great, trance is great, and depth is great. So, stop PM'ing me with your wisdom or I'm gonna' find out who you are and where you live and make up shit about you (yeah THAT kinda' shit!) and tell your parents. And they'll believe me because I'm an adult and adults wouldn't make shit up... okay?!

So where were we? Ahhhh yes, we relax them. I never met John Grinder, but I remember reading that in giving advice with a hypnotic subject he had advised: *"Relax the hell outta' them!"* I do hope he did say that. Because it's great advice. 'A relaxed subject is a relaxed subject' and waaaaaaay easier to work with. How do we do that? For me I do a *very standard* body relaxation from the feet to the head. I learned it in the early seventies.

It works perfectly hence I've never tried to mend it or change it. Remember that beautiful saying: *"If it ain't broke then stop buggering about with it!"*

Clip 8)...*YouTube:* Relaxation Clip

PART 10/16 RELEASE

So as I said earlier, I really believe that to be human is to be anxious, to a greater or lesser extent. And why wouldn't we? We live on a piece of earth that travels through space at a zillion miles an hour (okay so it's only 67,000 mph but that's still fast!) and all we can really do is hold on. We can't get away because of this thing called gravity although we've been as far as the moon (let's just say we have yeah?) and we're working towards Mars. It's funny how imprisonment can take place without one even being aware of it. I mean what are the chances we, human beings, potentially the most dangerous creatures in the universe have finally all been corralled up and placed here in this penal colony to safeguard the rest of the universe from us? It's got *my* vote! So yeah, they're hypnotised (maybe) and relaxed and now it's my job to *release them* of their problems in 3 areas, whether they have them or not! In my experience we nearly all carry them in some way.

And these are:

1) Anxiety

2) Worries (of the past, present and future)

3) Guilt, Shame and Remorse (we need to be careful how we phrase this one!)

(yes I am perfectly aware there are indeed a ton of other things but I believe that these cover most of the stuff they bring into the therapy room)

I say exactly this to every single client who sits in my chair for the first time:

"And now all I need you to do is simply allow, there goes that word again. I want you to allow all anxieties to leave your body…now. Simply drifting away from you, just like smoke, spiralling away from a small campfire, spiralling away, just getting higher and higher and higher till all of those anxieties … are quite simply… gone.

And now I want you to concentrate just for a moment on any and all worries you have ever had in the past, any and all worries you might be experiencing now, and any and all worries about your future…and again you simply allow all of those worries to simply drift…that's right… drift away from you… just like smoke…spiralling away from a campfire. Lifting higher…and higher…and higher… until they too are simply…gone.

And you know it's a funny thing, but every single human being who has ever lived, me included, has at some time

137

experienced some form… of guilt, shame or remorse. Real or imagined. Often unknown by they themselves! Sure, sometimes we do something wrong in life and yes, we feel guilty about that… but we hold our hands up, apologise and move on. However, a lot of the time we have nothing to actually be guilty about! We get blamed for things that were not actually our fault. We are made to feeeeeeel guilty, we are made to feel shame or remorse when we are actually not guilty. Yet often human beings take that on board!

(this can be quite a tense period in the session, where the client can become highly emotional, even to the point where abreactions can take place on a problem *unnamed* by the therapist, or even something which they themselves don't understand. It's simply a release of …stuff!)

So… if you have any of those feelings… of guilt, shame or remorse, recognise now that they are of no value to you… and you can now simply allow those feelings to simply float away from you, as I said, like smoke spiralling away from a campfire… getting higher… and higher… and higher till all those feelings go right up so high… they pass the clouds, moon, stars and go to the far end of the universe where they simply… disappear… leaving you feeling absolutely and completely…at ease. Totally at peace with yourself. And now you can just… breathe…….. relax…all the way down… feeling fantastic…"

Notice here in the last part how I DON'T say, "And knowing you, you'll be as guilty as hell for lots of stuff, am I right?" Guilt shame and remorse *must* be addressed. Because so many people do indeed carry these things but never want to talk about it and never really want to address it (at *this* point). So, our approach must be extremely tender and we really need to consider our wording, *'And you know it's a funny thing…' 'Every single human being (not just them)' 'me included'…'possibly real or imagined' 'unknown why'… 'not actually our fault'… 'made to feeeeeel guilty' etc*

And now that we have released and settled them, we can now address the problem.

PART 11/16   ADDRESS THE PROBLEM

Remember that this is a complete set of protocols on how to conduct an Initial Consultation and how to break down any walls. It is not an actual full teaching of any particular method. Yet I will happily claim that someone skilled in the art or rapport, by simply using The Wall will find that many of their clients will immediately have their anxieties and stresses lowered. However, let's have a look at addressing problems, shall we? So, if you the reader have the skills to look at and understand the methods within The Wall you will indeed see its therapeutic values and how we have now taken the client here, to this very special place where we can now use all that information they gave us at the beginning (in our notes), and simply by using that rapport I just mentioned, we can reframe all of it in order to help them in some way.

I'm a therapist. I want to help. However, … **this is where we find 'the standard script' sliding away to have a *mere* template put in its place.** Simply because it is here where we will find a whole smorgasbord of clients, all with *differing* problems and finding *different* ways of exhibiting those problems, therefore they themselves will be *different* to work with. We will still be using learned skills and some wording but there will be for example two main paths to travel upon at this point. And that will depend on the behaviour of the client during The Wall.

For example, you might find in your therapy room what we might term a total *somnambulist* with mild anxiety (don't we just pray for them?). In my experience we can just about *tell them* to stop feeling anxious and get a result!

Yet it has to said that there is a certain *fuddy-duddiness* within certain therapists who almost hate another therapist getting an easy fix. It's as though all treatment *has to be* highly technical and/or deeply scientific... and only something known by... *them!*

Back to the *HOW* and I wrote a moment ago there were two *main* paths to travel upon (although there are indeed several). If the first is the path in dealing with and treating a *somnambulist* then the second, by definition. is in dealing with and treating the *non-somnambulist*.

This is something (working with non-somnambulists who do not/cannot enter hypnosis) that can terrify newer hypnotherapists since all of their training is based on the belief from the training school that they are about to find their therapy rooms packed with these people who will be falling into hypnosis!

Anyhow... in the Initial Consultation this is my preferred default position. I use that term because quite often, mainly through The Swan I will already have made communication with a part within the subconscious (real or imagined) and have agreed on the method we are about to use. Indeed, possibly even been told it's being fixed *right now!*

But other than The Swan having already *told me* we *have a deal;* I personally will go for this form of addressing the problem as I simply wish to cover all the angles.

(in the early days of being a therapist I would find reasons *not to have to do*. Now I find reasons *to do*. I hope that makes sense).

But right now, I know that whether or not I am working with a somnambulist (who goes into hypnosis) or a non-somnambulist (who does not go into hypnosis) here's the deal… I don't care! All I need is for the part within the subconscious (or from anywhere really because *subconscious* is *only* a construct!) to accept and agree with either my argument or my request and… bingo! We are in with *waaaay* more than just a fighting chance. So yes, I'm saying…

"In a hypnotherapy room with a patient and a hypnotherapist, hypnotherapy does not need to take place in order for the patient to get fixed."

And what I've given you right there, is totally, completely and absolutely BETTER than anything *evidence based*. Rather it's a **FACT!!!** And anyone who tells you differently you need to run away from them!

So, once I have done the RELEASE, I then tell them to relax and remind them that earlier we agreed they don't have a problem. Not a conscious problem. If they had they would have fixed it themselves by now. Rather it's a subconscious problem which is totally inside them, yet totally outside their control...

"So now I want you to relax even deeper into your chair as you tune into my voice. Just the timbre of my voice. Don't fight me but don't try and help me. Your job remember... is to do nothing. And simply allow me to go talk to that part inside you who knows exactly what's going on..."

Now at this point I maybe have been given (during The Swan) a name from that part inside. It's maybe Jimmy or Angela or Mum or Grandad or Vangoosha from the planet Mantach... whatever The Swan told me. Or I didn't get a name just a good contact. Or I didn't get a good contact, just good response tests. Or I didn't get good response tests, but they did relax very well. Or they didn't relax very well but they seemed to slip into hypnosis on the induction. Or they definitely did not go into hypnosis and they were no good whilst Swanning...etc.

All of those might tweak me into a different type of approach, however, lets choose one of the most difficult. A worst-case scenario if you will?

And I absolutely love worse case scenarios. Because it's there where I get some of my best results! Which of course is both wonderful and at times bloody annoying.

So, with this client, let's call her Jane. She has challenges walking the dog at night. Going shopping. Attending parties with her husband. Even walking into a room where there are people already there. I think I can safely say I will work with hundreds of these type of clients every year but in this case we shall assume she was not a good responder either during The Swan or at any other stage in The Consultation. Basically, she was only good at closing her eyes when I asked her to.

But this is indeed a great case for you guys to look at. Especially if you are fairly new to this field. Because in a way this is how therapy works or can work very often. I have not much to go on *with Jane*. But I do have lots to go on *with this type of case.* I have been here many, many times. I have walked through this swamp. I know where the loose stones are and where the deepest mud is.

There is a saying that *if you don't know what the hell you're doing then you need to make something up.* If I'm being candid, I do believe that over the earlier years in certain situation where my training and skills were obviously *not working* that's exactly what I did. Then I sharpened my skills and got better. Then I got some great results which were repeated. Then I travelled the world and through my work I now know at least many hundreds of therapists from all over whom I get to check my facts with on a regular basis.

But alas, very often we get told that our work is merely of an anecdotal nature as opposed to evidence based, Although I was pretty convinced that I had an idea I looked up 'anecdotal' several years ago to be sure what my scientific colleagues were saying about me and my work. I wrote it down. Here it is:

'Anecdotal evidence is evidence from anecdotes (anecdote: a short amusing or interesting story) stories, evidence collected in a casual or informal manner and relying heavily or entirely on personal testimony.*

So there y'go!

I read an evidence based story recently about two guys who sounded like Phillngton and Jewsonberry who had been to Oxford and Cambridge and had degrees and stuff and had something in an article in a psychological journal of how they had ran a test on 73 people and had gotten a high percentage result of something like 60 out of the 73 which meant that this test was now **evidence based**, even though it had failed 20% of the time, and I thought:

"Well bugger me! So evidence based is far worse than anything I have ever achieved with my anecdotal healings! Wow!"

Anyway, we're not scientists. we're better than that. we're therapists. I'm not a scientist. I'm a clinical hypnotist. And I've never met a scientist or evidence-based therapist who gets better results than me or any other of my colleagues *in the therapy room*. So, what's a boy to do? But neither I nor anyone else can tell another person how to *address the problem* in either a sentence or a chapter or a book. There are just too many paths containing too many possibilities. However, as crazy as it sounds, when it comes to addressing the problem of the client sitting across from me m*y* notes tell me what to do! I have been writing almost non-stop throughout the entire consultation. I have a good hold on their problem by now and you will remember the question I asked them prior to placing them into hypnosis? Here it is again, *"So just as a matter of interest, if I had a magic wand and I could wave it in the air in order for you to know that something had happened today, that you would know a change had taken place, what would that be?"*

This is my very favourite question I ask throughout the entire consultation. And that, coupled with all the information I have about them tells me exactly where to go. So yes, in addressing their actual problem I will always attempt at this point to make contact with 'the part within the subconscious' (rather than the subconscious itself!) and IF contact does get made I will ask the simple question, *"Can we make something happen... today?"* Then I see what happens. Why go with something *imagined* when you can go with something, potentially *real* or imagined?

And yes of course I know that many will look upon me as if I'm an idiot in saying that, but I have literally hundreds of fellow **Swanners** whom I know well and who will be smiling as they read this. Nobody ever said we can't have fun in the therapy room whilst discovering *other* realities. And as **Swanners** we are totally aware of other realities!

So in addressing the problem I *go talk to the guy.* I try to find out who's in charge, always by saying thank you for the things they have done for this person who will most likely not be aware that anything has *ever* been done for them. And then acknowledging things had to happen for a reason BUT...putting forward a philosophical argument that, maybe it's time? Maybe it's time for change. Here of course if it's pain I give thanks for the message but now argue for either:

a) a possible fix (why not? I cannot think of *one single thing* to lose by going for that!) b) a reduction in the pain, or perhaps a heat or warm glow to take its place. Remember that pain is a message. But unlike other earthlings, human beings for some reason appear to embrace that message too tightly. We need to slacken that hold!

c) the possibility of beginning to work together in healing whilst pain is reduced

I always end *Addressing The Problem* by suggesting happiness, confidence, strength etc to swim through their entire being, as all good hypnotists should... like I said whether they're in 'what we call' hypnosis or not!

And in repeating much of my wording I get to witness head nods, huge breaths, emotion, smiles, laugher even as I use my art-form to weave for my client some... Pavlovian magic! Erm... I hope that rings a bell for some of you, yes?

(trust me that is very *very* clever *and* funny! ☺)

PART 12/16   INSERT IMPREGNABLE BUBBLE

As already said a good idea doesn't care who uses it, and this idea was certainly not originally mine. Back in 1982 I trained with the Jose Silva Group and was impressed with a technique they had called *The Impregnable Bubble*. I now use it in every case I have. The client simply allows all the bad stuff to leave and of course I have inserted all the good stuff (after addressing the problem). I use it for the simple reason that many of these people that we fix quite simply don't stay fixed as that problem, physical or mental, can very easily return. A skilled therapist understands this and looks out for it. Life happens. And when that takes place the therapist will most probably not *be* there. Therefore, I love the idea of the client having something that I have either given or taught them. Something which they themselves can use. And of course, you the therapist can add whatever you have been talking about with your client, prestige, confidence, courage, confidence etc, before closing and sealing this invisible impregnable bubble.

But you know what? I learned over the years that there were clients who I did a fantastic job with and they left feeling fantastic! The impregnable bubble was in place.....but.... suddenly there would be a kinda' *fly-by* of the old thought or thoughts. The old programme. And sometimes when that happened they, the client, would frame this as, *"It's here again! That can only mean... that the treatment didn't work. It's back!"* So we needed something on top of that!

PART 13/16... BLOWAWAY TECHNIQUE

So, we have ran a great session and we have inserted The Impregnable Bubble to ensure all the bad stuff is out and all the good stuff is in. All is just about perfect, until, the *Moon, Junes and Ferris Wheels* of the lovely songwriter Joni Mitchell turn up. Clouds get in the way! So, after inserting The Impregnable Bubble we say,

".... now I need you to remember that although you are lying there in a nice relaxed state, where we have successfully done some hypnosis, but we haven't taken away any of your thoughts or memories. And strangely enough every so often you might feel just a hint of those old feelings swimming around...outside that bubble perhaps... but here's the thing... you need to know that they are just memories. Old memories flying by. They don't even need to be acknowledged. They are just echoes. Echoes of thoughts that used to be. And if that should ever happen, we just allow them to pass by on their way... OR we can actually

help them on their way… we simply take care of those echoes. We do that by taking a deep breath... all the way in... (it's not imperative, however I myself personally pace this, in order to see if the client actually takes that deep breath in)... *and we simply blow it away* (the therapist blows) *and guess what? We can even laugh at ourselves* (said laughingly) *for being crazy enough to do this! We simply take a deep breath in.... and we blow! That's right…that's right!"* Thankyou Milt [private joke just for therapists ☺].

And of course in doing this you'll either get complete silence with no movement, or some heavy breathing or in many cases they will indeed take in huge breaths and blow all over the room, revealing the reality they are experiencing at the time.

PART 14/16... CONFIRMATION (if possible)

So, as you can see, after hypnosis and/or relaxing our client, we Address the Actual Problem *before* inserting the Impregnable Bubble along with The Blowaway Technique. However, although we cannot be sure of an actual *fix*, at this time, it is important that we be brave enough to 'test our work'. By that I mean that we can at the very least *ask* the part within the subconscious if it is with us. Remembering of course that the subconscious might very well be with us but not able to create any form of IMR or voice confirmation. But it's important to at least *go there* and *see* what happens. At this point in time the therapist can put the client's arm into the shape of The Swan, or go for IMR's in their preferred style (finger twitch or a raised arm), or even go for **Direct Voice from The Swan...**

Direct Voice is where we talk to the part controlling the sitter's hand and simply say: "If you can control their finger and hand and arm do you think it's possible that you can also control their cardiovascular system? Their heart, lungs, voice box and simply say: *'Hello'?"...* and we then wait for the part, real or imagined to talk to us, often going into very deep discussion, in order to get confirmation that all of this has been done and will be worked upon even more strongly over the coming week. So, what I'm talking about here is openly asking the part/subconscious/higher self/guide/entity within the client to confirm that your work is answered. That the magic has taken place. And to give confirmation with any of the above.

TRUTH MOMENT!!!!!!!!!!!!!!!! (Not too many trainers or fellow therapists wish to admit this, but all over the world excellent therapists will get that sign of confirmation and yet... a) the client will NOT be healed! or b) no sign of confirmation will be given and yet they are fixed for life! As the saying goes, *"When the magic doesn't work, we use therapy"* So... welcome to the world of therapy. But seriously it's a reminder that this is not mathematics. This is a soft science for sure but hypnotherapy is also an art. And in hypnotherapy, 'the mathematician and scientist will very often struggle whilst the artist wins' (Bob Burns 2020).... Ooooh but I do hope I get quoted on that! ☺
But this is the deal, yeah? We check our work.

PART 15/16... EXPLAIN SESSIONS

Fairly straightforward yes? You simply explain to the client how you normally run your business and what you think might be best for them next. Personally, I suggest the client may wish to go home, see how they feel and let me know if they wish to come back for further sessions. I am quite happy to inform the client that most people see me for between 3 or 4 sessions. However, in approximately 90% of these initial sessions the client wishes to book another session there and then.

Part 16/16... NOTES (including hypnotic rating)

I personally go through my notes after each session and log them immediately. My mind at this point in time is fresh, both in my knowledge of them and ideas for the next session. I also have a note of where I see each of my clients on the hypnotic scale of 1-10. And yes, I always test each client for skills in hypnotic skills during the initial consultation. If *you* don't do that you simply cannot *be* a hypnotherapist.

Phew! This has been a hard CHAPTER for you. I'm not sure if you could actually find any enjoyment in it. But I can only say that all of the above is entirely factual. This is what I do. And I get excellent results. I do hope with the added online clips I have somehow given you a measure of the *feel* in my therapy room. And one day you might even join me there. There is a lot of laughter in my therapy room, especially in the initial consultation, and my students (who normally become my friends) speak well of me I believe (since most of my work is through personal recommendation) and, more importantly, they get to see and remember the results they have witnessed in my therapy room. At this time of writing I have been <u>training people in the therapy room</u> for around 20 years or so. And I personally have never met anyone else in the world that trains in this way. I have simply no real idea why that is. What instructor/tutor/teacher would not have a strong desire to reveal to their student how the skill actually works in real time with real people in the arena where it all takes place? And yes here in 2021 I now mentor people who are allowed to watch me work live with clients on line. A couple small caveats on that. If it's of a sexual nature I do not take a third person into the therapy room with me, and if it gets fairly deep and tense I will ask that third person to leave the room. It's only happened once however.

CHAPTER 9

Authoratative versus Permissive

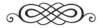

I know many suggestive authoritarian hypnotists, indeed some of them are my good friends who are fantastic in purely suggestive hypnosis with an authoritarian style that TELLS the subject exactly what to do. And I'm happy to believe that more often than not they will be able to create minor miracles right there in the therapy room. However, for me, that would be the kind of approach I would take whilst hypnotising someone commercially in a stage show or whilst doing magic or mentalism say, or just for fun at a dinner party or maybe doing 'street hypnosis' as I hang out *'wid my bros'* (Yeah I'm of the street, so sue me).

In these situations, I want to move fast and I want to enjoy it. I always want to suggest to my audience that I have some kind of strange esoteric power enough to make them go, "ooooooh!" all linked to my ego of course. I have discovered over the years that many of my colleagues are incredibly deep thinkers whilst I find that due to my commercial and entertainment background perhaps (?) I can indeed be ridiculously shallow! ☹ The message is that hypnosis can *be* fun and nobody ever needs to get embarrassed in any way. Many of the very best hypnotists in the world are also great hypnotees and they love to volunteer *themselves.* But of course, authoritarian hypnosis can be used in the therapy room if and when required. Indeed in the therapy room, if I'm being honest, every so often I will often pick up on something said or a gesture or statement or twitch or look that will guide me into suddenly doing an instant induction where I find myself being extremely authoritarian and just telling the client very directly to *"sleep!"* And indeed, I have very often told my subject to very simply, *"stop it!"* In fact, this is an in joke used by many hypnotherapists paying homage to that beautiful clip by Bob Newhart.

In his show (The Newhart Show) he played a Chicago psychologist (Robert Hartlet) where he put together the "Stop It!" skit, which although being highly funny had hundreds of skilled therapists right across the world who, whilst becoming aware of the brilliant comedy mind of Bob Newhart, also recognised something, which I'm sure Mr Newhart himself had no idea about when he wrote his skit. Because at the end of the day if we can say and get an agreement on *"Stop it, stop it now!"* then strangely enough it can indeed become a done deal! .... and there is *a chance* of the magic taking place instantly! Although the skilled therapist knows that most likely a few more sessions might be needed to solidify and support the session.

This is something reported in hundreds of cases, which again begs the questions, WHO and WHAT *are* we?).

Clip 9)...*YouTube:* Stop it! - (Bob Newhart skit)

But for me, in the therapy room I am certainly not an authoritative hypnotist. I think I'd be best described as a permissive therapist. I use please and thankyou a lot when I am talking to those parts within the patient but yes, I can turn from good cop into bad cop when I need to, (this is an exaggeration of course and apologies to all authoritative hypnotherapists ☺). Just as a matter of interest, although there are the normal assumed differences between what we consider to be permissive hypnotherapists, as one who seeks permission to do something, normally perhaps in a pleasing way whilst the authoritative method sometimes appears to be that of power. Perhaps quite commanding and almost demanding respect and an insistence on being obeyed. However, it's interesting to look at where this word authoritative comes from. And basically, we are looking to *the opinion of the author* where a certain piece of work is thought of as being authoritative. Arguably the author has the absolute and final word on the matter. No one else's opinion matters. Not the publisher, not the printer, not the critic, not even the reader because only the author truly knows where the work comes from. Oocha' boy! As I said, arguable but it reveals where that *authoritative stance* might have its roots? ☺

There is a lovely story from a friend of mine and excellent clinical hypnotist Barry Thain (Mindsci Clinical Hypnotherapy, Richmond, Surrey) where he suggested in a forum that with a very good hypnotee it should be at least possible that if the subject was scared of bees then all you would have to do would be to get him or her to close their eyes and the tell them, *"Bees are cute. One two... eyes open wide awake!"* and then ask them how they felt about bees only to be told "Bees are cute!" Now let me make this perfectly clear, Barry would not have actually delivered this kind of therapy I'm sure, as he is an extremely responsible therapist. Rather he was (quite comedically I thought) demonstrating what might possibly happen, perhaps with a great subject. But I remember when I read his post thinking, *"Yeah, maybe!"*. Indeed, I liked his example so much that, just for fun I put it to the test one day! I had helped arrange a one-day workshop for Freddy and Anthony Jacquin (United Kingdom Hypnotherapy Training College) at a very nice venue in Stirlingshire. I was attending with a good friend of mine and a great stage hypnotist from Arbroath, Andy Lawson. Just before we were breaking for tea that morning, I had been partnered up during the workshop with a young man who, just by pure coincidence at the very end happened to mention to me his morbid fear of bees. It was one of those moments where a statement prompts a thought. It was kinda' like a sign, and I honestly remember thinking to myself, thinking back to what Barry Thain had said, *"I'm gonna' DO this!"* as I just simply asked him, if I could show him a way to get rid of that fear forever, would he be interested? To which he said he'd be delighted. So, I got him to close his eyes. Then literally *told* him *"Bees are cute. One, two, wide awake!"*, exactly like that as I wanted to literally copy the wording that Barry had used in his post several months earlier. He opened his eyes and I asked him, as if it were for the very first time, how he felt about bees and he told me that he actually found them to be rather cute! I simply laughed and walked up to the bar for a coffee, to be honest whispering the F word under my breath. Sure, that was interesting. But the really interesting thing happened *next*. After about 10 mins I was approached by Derek Heron, an excellent professional mentalist based in Hamilton in Scotland, who was attending that day. I do believe Derek said something like, *"You'd better get your arse out there Bob!"* ... and when I looked through the window there was my boy standing in a huge bush... covered with bees and looking totally delighted with himself!

So, I get out there, being watched now by a fairly fascinated audience, and quite timidly enter the bush, talking to my man gently and persuading him that we really should step back out *away* from the bees. Which of course was so difficult since he truly did find them *soooooo* cute! And the crazy thing was that he was fine, not a mark on him, whilst I got stung twice taking him away from his friends in the bush! Do you think the bees knew something? 😊 When I got him back inside, we did all the right things this time. I popped him back under before allowing his fears to be gone and the fascination with these lovely earth-saving creatures to remain. *But...* no longer would he attempt to enter bushes and try to pet them! Rather he would allow them to get on with their lives in perfect harmony.

So yes, this does remind me of the power in authoritative hypnosis. Where with a good client, miracles can indeed happen right there and then. But you need to BE the hypnotist (I cannot suggest strongly enough that you pause for a moment and take that last sentence *in*!).

I want if I may at this time to mention a wonderful hypnotist who has now passed away, the late Jeffrey Stephens. Since his passing his number one student and a good former student and now friend of mine, Rob de Groof now teaches Jeff's methods over in Belgium. I learned a great deal from Jeff and I remember discussing what would be the best method of doing this thing we call hypnotherapy. Jeff favoured the authoritative style whilst I preferred the permissive. Whilst we both of course recognised that it would depend on the skill of the individual therapists when presenting either. Jeff's argument was that the authoritative style simply worked better, and I guess watching *his* style and *his* skill set I could not give him an argument on that. But my mind was on training a mass of people where we need to be more sure on what the better approach might be? Having said that I do believe Jeff understood that but still would have preferred the authoritative style, *(at this time of writing I spoke to Rob de Groof who now teaches Jeff's method around the world and he agrees with Jeff LOL. In all fairness I do believe Jeff was Rob's first tutor.)* But for me I was reminded of the good cop/bad cop. It is a great psychological *kinda'* protocol used in interrogating a suspect where both styles are laid at the door, where strangely enough either can actually work. But it is recognised as doubling the chances of getting the suspect to comply and tell the truth of course.

My argument was simply based on my findings (*all* of my arguments are based on my findings), which you the reader may very well disagree with and that's fine. But I found that if I start a procedure as a permissive therapist it normally works better.

but if it is not working, I can abruptly change to being authorative (kinda' like good cop to bad cop?) and get a really good result BECAUSE of that change. However, (**and this is extremely important**) I discovered over many years, that if I go in authoritatively and *do not get a result* it's almost as if I have 'shown my hand'? It's almost as if that part/entity/angel/guide/fairy/spaceman (real or imagined) looks at me and says, *"too late. I've already seen who you really are. And now you're merely pretending to be nice."*

And like I said, my findings have shown time and time again that I can indeed get a result when good cop suddenly turns into bad cop. But when bad cop tries to be good cop it totally throws the part into disarray. So, why go in with only one chance when you can have two? 😊 *(remember? Snekarios Estas Bestas!)* But sometimes of course it doesn't really matter that much whether your authoritative, permissive, or any other style. Sometimes all the best work you do seems to work but doesn't. In my particular style of work using my particular protocols I am keen to use a permissive style in order to use The Swan, through consultation (The Wall) in order to get an agreed consensus, from a part, which I accept as real or imagined, that the job will get done.

But sometimes, that doesn't quite take place...

CHAPTER 10

The Battleship

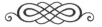

A part of my training in managing people was that whether I liked it or not there would be times when I had to *be the monster they needed at that time*. Yes I do know that that will make a few readers twitch in considering that to be quite reprehensible, but… stop it! Stop it now!!!

I can say that was one of the best teachings handed down to me, I was told that at these times I was not give them my reasons, rather I had to give them my decisions. And that was because they'd never understand my reasons, whilst they would at least always understand my decisions. Again I found this to be absolutely brilliant advice. And in the therapy room at times I use this advice for the benefit of the client.

It's lovely to be able to have the skills to do all the jolly things a hypnotist can do, give them amnesia, stick them to chairs, get them to think your invisible etc. And all of these things in the hand of a good therapist aren't just games. They really can be important as convincers before the work actually begins. If I can get them to forget their name then I can get them to forget their problem… if I can stick them to the chair then I can stick them to their goal… if I can make myself seem invisible than I can also make the problem seem invisible… Most of the above of course will in the main be short term. By that I mean that more *real* work will normally be required when we address not just the effect but rather the cause. Although it doesn't *have* to be that way. The hypnotic therapy room truly can be a place where miracles can indeed seem very real. However, when I am doing workshops or mentoring in my therapy room, I often get asked the question with regard to: *"After you have performed all the magic... is it guaranteed to work?"*

And of course the honest answer is a firm NO unless you are one of those nutcase therapists who claim they, a) fix everyone and b) they do it in one session. Hey a couple of them are friends of mine! But *no* it's not a problem. Rather it becomes a pretty decent challenge that needs attending to.

Now we therapists are all different. However in MY world where I communicate with a third party, real or imagined, inside the client, I need to know what I do next if we (the communicating part and I) have initially agreed on a good outcome, and that good outcome does *not* happen. So, here we have it, the next session where a linked part (real or imagined) within the client has promised to stop the problematic activity or pain or feelings in order that we get together in a week and see if we can totally resolve the issue pleasing all parties (or PARTS). You may remember earlier I was talking about good cop and bad cop? I like to keep an ace up my sleeve, and that ace can very often be that bad cop. Or if you like, quite simply, the one that is not interested in negotiating (because we tried that?), but rather TELLS the client/part exactly what to do! This is indeed my whole argument with authoritative hypnosis compared to permissive therapy. If you're a *good* cop you can change at any given time, as you will see... but if you reveal yourself initially as the *bad* cop, then it's very difficult to try and change and get *the part* on your side. You have indeed as they say, *shot your bolt.* This is why I developed this particular protocol. It's for when a part within the client tells me, promises me, that it/they will guarantee that a certain thing will happen and it does not! This is how I handle the next session, This is The Battleship Protocol:

The client is sitting across from me, and has just given me the message that, despite receiving confirmation last week from the part/person/guide/energy, that there would be a huge change... there has been *none*! So, after all the magic, a truly fantastic session which the client themselves saw as confirmation nothing has actually changed. So, we need to find out why,

After relaxing the client, I elicit the part to acknowledge it is here in the room (normally through The Swan). I then welcome them, thank them for returning and say how wonderful it is to meet them again. Then I tell them I have a question I wonder if they'd be good enough to answer for me.

And then... I BANG my fist as hard as I can on the table (they *always* jump!) and exclaim in a *very* load voice: *"WHAT part of I promise did you not understand?!"*
And although nothing actually happens at this point the tension in the room is palpable. Then I ask... very slowly...
"Do...YOU...hear...me...?"

I will nearly ALWAYS get a yes response at this point. I go on...

"Perhaps I didn't explain this properly... Y'see...we are on a ship... But it's not a passenger ship... It's not a cruiseship...

161

And we are not allowing any stowaways... THIS... is a BATTLESHIP! (another SLAP on the word BATTLESHIP). *Do...you...understand?"*

The question is mainly rhetorical but often at this point I will get a strong *yes*.

Now, you need to understand that we are at WAR. We, you and I, are doing every...single...thing... that we can... in order to save...NAME OF CLIENT... and I need you right HERE...by my side... Do...you...understand... that? Now if you can help that's fine, if not I will talk to a different part that can help!!! But I need you to lead from the front or help from the side or get the hell out of the way. Do you understand THAT? Can you DO that? Are you HAPPY to DO that? Can I COUNT on you (these questions will mostly receive huge yes answers)*?! Now then... what can you actually do? Let's talk..."*

I can honestly answer that I have never failed to get THE PART on my side at this point. Or at worst to *be* on my side whilst I become aware of another challenge out-with this situation (welcome to therapy). In other words, I get told a story that it could not keep the promise because of someone or thing. There are of course rebuttals we can use against argumentative parts, such as, *"YOU must be sick to death of this" "Isn't it time YOU got a change?"..."We need you here, and NOW, can we count on you?"..."You have been doing great but now we desperately need you to do THIS!"* However, guess what? Simply by the very USE of The Battleship Protocol I promise you that the problem kinda' gets knocked off its feet? IT...HE...SHE... truly gets MOTIVATED! But....... YOU have to

BE that person in the room when YOU are called upon.
Be ready. Be Brave. Be the person the client is praying you are!
Again... BE the hypnotist! Let's have a wee look at this in action,
shall we?

Clip 10... *YouTube:* BATTLESHIP DEMONSTRATION

But, y'know, there are indeed certain times, certain strange
times when you're just totally NOT in control! It's like there's a
'glitch in The Matrix'! Let's have a look at such a situation in our
next CHAPTER (just try not to enjoy it too much okay?) and see
how fate sometimes steps into our life and... kinda' screws us?

CHAPTER 11

Buddy – A Salutary Tale

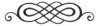

(Every career should have a life-changing moment. This one was mine)

I'm happy to tell this story not just because it's kinda' funny but it also reveals something of the hypnotic state and what can happen within it. Hypnosis can be many things. A deep state approaching sleep, to a mild slumber, to being totally wide awake with eyes completely open. And sometimes a form of sleep accompanied by a truly incredible form of awareness. I guess we all have some interesting or strange stories of things that happened to us that simply could never be written by any writer. Anyway it's probably time I went public with this one, My friends and family know that I have been involved in all kinds of healing since my twenties and as anyone who has ever been involved in any form whatsoever of alternative healing, we find, do we not, that at certain times, regardless of the fact we don't have the time or we can't really see where we can help in that particular situation, that it is almost impossible to keep our mouths.....shut?! We just *have* to offer our help. And so, it was that I found myself one afternoon in one of Hampshire's lovely railway towns, Eastleigh. It was a little after 2.00.p.m and I had entered a hairdressers to ask some information and there she stood, this lovely wee lady with a beautiful smile. And yet bent shoulders, a furrowed brow. It was the eyes that really told her story. They were sunk well into her head and there was discolouring in the skin below. She hadn't been sleeping and actually seemed a bit teary. I simply couldn't stop my mouth from talking, *"I hope you don't mind me asking but are you in a LOT of pain?"* She went on to inform me that she was a sufferer of the dreaded arthritis and that today had been a particularly bad day for her. We don't know how it happens do we? I am involved in the healing arts and I wouldn't want it any other way, but my wife is forever telling me that my mouth gets me into trouble, I don't quite know how to say no, or even that I need a moment. But that's how it works isn't it? Our mouths open and we simply say it. In my case it came across as something like:

"Wow, I'm sorry to hear that. Listen, I am very aware that we have never met, but sometimes... well, sometimes I'm able to help people who are in pain."

We then covered the fact that I wasn't a doctor and that I didn't charge for this service, which is often a worrying thought since it baffles people as to why people like us exist! What's IN IT for US?! But there she was in a lot of pain and ready to seek help anywhere, and there was me. The problem was she had people to see and would not be free until 6.00.p.m. And as crazy as it sounds, she then gave me her private address and directions on how to get there along with the explanation that she and her husband would be there at that time and how he was 'a little bit funny about stuff like this'. 'Perfect' I thought to myself. All the ingredients were there to ensure an absolute car-crash. My English wife has spent many years warning me about situations not to get into, based on situations I've previously gotten into. She has a certain look. It's simply a very slow head shake. I often imagine her and that look when I get into trouble. I even tell her later, when I get into trouble that I was angry with her for giving me that look. Although she wasn't actually there and she didn't know *I* was there, but I know she would have given me that look when I get *unlucky* in situations, and it makes me angry with her? C'mon! There must be many people out there who understand this? Okay maybe a couple? Right one then, there must be *one* of you for chrissakes??!!

Anyway, I got to her home early. I was based along the road in Southampton, which was less than 5 miles away. 90 mins drive in the rush hour. They finally drew up 45 minutes late which was not a problem. I mean if you ask anyone who does pro-bono work for human beings, they will happily inform you that they get *shat upon* on a regular basis. It's strange I know but there it is! They leave the car and the husband (string vest and working men's cords) glowers at me angrily. I'm obviously interfering with his supper. I mumble something about rhubarb (I can't remember why, it's all part of my ADHD stuff I think) and we walk to the door. The lady looks worse than she did earlier. We enter the family home and there he is, **Buddy!** The biggest blackest strongest Labrador I have ever seen. String Vest drags Buddy away from me and sits on the main chair as I sit next to his wife on the sofa. I mumble some stuff sycophantly in explanation of what I do, how it's part healing and part hypnosis perhaps and yaddyaddyaddy.... Everything is going averagely well until she turns to her husband and asks if it could be possible for him and Buddy to go upstairs while I try to help her.

He lets go of a few expletives and slams the door behind him. I'm not going to try to make this all mystical or esoteric, but whether it's a hypnotist, healer, mentalist, magician, NLP'er or any kind of artist about to do their work, it is so important to be 'in the zone'. To have a moment. To be calm in order to gather your thoughts, emotions, energies etc and right at that moment I was a bit Harpo Marx-ist. But we go on. I always ask someone in pain if they could give me a number from one to ten to give me an idea of how bad their pain is what would that be? The lady reported a solid nine. I decided to do a straight hypnotic induction, as it saves time with healing techniques which have been lain down for centuries. Then we'd see where we were. The problem being of course getting the lady into state (assuming there is such a thing). I got lucky, she was a great somnambulist and although she told me she had never been hypnotised before she went *boing* immediately. A dream to work with for any hypnotist and I already had a strong expectancy that my work would be beneficial, and hopefully now that I knew how she worked I could refer her to someone I might know in the area for future help after I had long gone. It was going spiffingly well until suddenly I heard the heavily padded noise coming down the stairs. It didn't sound like human feet. And when the door opened slowly (don't ask me how) and I saw Buddy's wet black nose enter the room I thought to myself, as hypnotists and healers do, *"Aye aye, this might go tits up".* And so it was that he entered and walked in a long circle around the room gazing at me and licking his lips. At one point I swear I saw a smile spread across his salivating mouth. Anyway, I simply continued...

".... and any noises outside or even inside the room will only allow you to slip even deeper into that wonderful grandmother's feathered bed as you drift and dream and float..." God but I'm a good hypnotist! And although she was sitting her shoulders sagged even further as I performed The Cascade (a deepener) and she went even further into a beautiful relaxed state. It was then that Buddy decided to very slowly but boldly walk straight up to where I was sitting and then, beginning with his front paws and very decorously followed by his hind legs had now gotten himself up onto the sofa and was standing behind me. So, we had the situations of my good lady slumped but sitting on my left with her head flopped to her right almost resting on my shoulder. Me sitting next to and half-facing her and Buddy behind me on my right and starting to make a whining noise. It was a hypnotist friend of mine, Michael Skirving, who first said to me, *"They never bring their personal manual in with them. They don't have one. Therefore, we first have to find out how they work, in order for us to work on them."* And sadly, that is totally true. And not just of our patients. Buddy hadn't brought his manual in with *him* that evening. If he had I would have known that that whining noise was actually.... the mating call of a ten stone (bout' 140 pounds in American) three-year-old Labrador in love with a Scotsman (hey it happens)! Buddy began his courtship by placing his left paw on my left shoulder, then his right paw on my right shoulder. I whispered to him out the side of my mouth to desist but Buddy was quite recalcitrant (I know it's a big word for many of you but hey I'm writing a book here?). When the two paws came around the front and crossed each other around my

168

neck I knew how General Custer might have felt in his last minutes at Little Bighorn. It's difficult to explain exactly what happened next. I suddenly became a highly frantic plate spinner desperately trying to control *all* of my thoughts, whilst at the same time considering all the different scenarios that might unfold within the next 30 seconds or so. Obviously you would advise that the thing to do in that moment would be to stop having sex with Buddy, the ten stone (still about 140 pounds in American) Labrador and I promise you I totally appreciate that, however I had my art to consider. I had this woman in a trance state and I was responsible for her well-being... dammit! Then of course there would be the string-vest to think about. Should he ever become aware that the stranger downstairs was holding his wife (she was slumping towards me now) whilst having sex with his dog that might not augur well in developing a referral basis within the local community. And then, with Buddy hammering away at my spine (Thank Cheeeeeerist he had apparently no knowledge of human anatomy!) things took a turn for the worse. I kid you not when I say he put his chin on my right shoulder and his face pushed against mine, his mouth frothing a salacious smile at me and his eyes rolling upwards as his amygdala exploded, as you do. And although I appreciate that it was only in my imagination, I could clearly see my English wife, Leigh, standing in the corner of the room. Her arms crossed and that head of hers once again slooooowly shaking left and right, which again made me very angry with her! I felt that she was letting me down in her refusal to understand the situation fully?

All this time of course I am forever being the consummate professional, *"That's right, just drifting away as you just let all of that pain float away from you just like……. etc"* And then something happened. Understand what I said earlier, in that hypnosis is not simply hypnosis. It has many threads, ways, methods, modes, situations, conditions, processes, states and just when you think you know them all... you don't. I have absolutely no doubt in any way shape or form that the lady was in a profound state of what we would term hypnosis. But then this happened, she sat up, turned, opened her eyes, lifted her left hand and slapped Buddy hard in the face as she screamed, *"Leave him!"* ... before immediately closing her eyes and falling back into my arms. Well, we're now talking *shit and fans* here! Buddy let out a howl in a way that could never be described as mellifluous and jumped off the sofa and ran hiding under the table. Saved. Well... nearly! What with the lady screaming and the dog howling *string vest* now came thudding down the stairs and kicked open the door before turning to stare at me, *"What the fuck is going on mister?"*

I was simply fantastic. I looked totally puzzled, doing that thing with the wrinkled downturned Robert De Niro mouth and shook my head vigorously as I denied that we had heard any sounds here in the living room. Although when I said "nothing" I distinctly remember thinking I sounded more like Pasquale (hi-pitched English comedian) than De Niro.

String vest scratched his head and stared at the terrified Buddy cowering under the table as I woke the lady up. On asking her what number her pain was now at she answered that it was a one but that it wasn't really a pain, more of a warmth, which is quite a common reaction and something all experienced pain therapists will of course recognise. Then to make it even more ridiculous string-vest, on hearing how well his wife was, appeared to be not just placated but decided that he, just like Buddy, was also in love with me. He informed me of a pain in his foot and asked if I'd take a look at it. I suggested he allow the doctor to have a look at it first and then, only if the doctor could not help, he might want to consider pulling in someone like me. All the usual stuff happened with the lady being grateful and me suggesting that because she was such a good subject, although I would not be in the area again, I would happily recommend another therapist. And of course, Buddy looked devastated as I turned to leave. However, I gave him one solitary wink and mouthed 'I'll be back' and his tail went thud, just the once, against the carpet.

Anyway, it all ended well. Nobody said we can't have fun whilst doing therapy, eh? ☺

Chapter 12

A Flock of Swans

I literally have no idea how many testimonials and stories have been sent to me over the years from hypnotherapists, psychotherapists, psychologists, spiritual, psychic and energy healers and as you will see some of the very best professional mentalists in the world today. But it will definitely be well into the thousands. For me they are all beautiful and each one makes me smile *(thankyou, seriously!)*.

I am always aware and indeed touched that someone somewhere, most of the time a stranger, has taken time out of their life to touch my life. To tell me of how a little bit of my life touched theirs. These are *moments*. And for me they are indeed precious moments. So I thought that although it would obviously be too much to throw several thousand testimonials at you, it would be a good idea to simply pull out, totally at random I promise, some of these moments. Understand these testimonials/stories are untouched. I decided NOT to explain WHO the writers are. If you need to know you can find out. And no doubt some of you will indeed recognise some of them. Anyway, here they are (thankyou guys!)…

WAYNE TRICE (hypnotist and magician)
Want to say a huge thank you to Bob Burns for his Swan technique! Fantastic way into the subconscious. Actually, even

better it works on my 8-year-old! I had the DVD on, and he was getting bored listening to Bob discuss it (sorry Bob) and then the explanation came and he tried it and it worked. His face was a picture, he now asks me to talk to his subconscious.

MOSES (pro mentalist)

I performed this earlier this week and had a reaction I never had before-- it's something that Bob deals within his video (The Swan) but I had never experienced it personally before. I began the first phase and the person that I was doing this with freaked out when things began to happen. She turned her head away and couldn't watch-- but the Swan kept on swimming along. I appreciate that you put that particular participant on the DVD, Bob, it allowed me to handle the moment as a fun one instead of a potentially stressful one. I love this more and more!

SETH SPEAKS (pro mentalist)

I have finally had a chance to watch this, and it is elegant and wonderful. I'm absolutely staggered. Bob Burns has a *terrific* teaching style, an incredible voice and manner, and he makes it seem so easy. I'm very thankful to have this in my toolkit. Thanks so much, Bob!!! Seth

LUCA VOLPE (pro mentalist, Italy)

This is powerful stuff! Elegant and poetic! Is a great pleasure to finally know Bob too! Thanks for this release! Pablo Amira (pro mentalist) An absolutely wonderful, artistic and beautifully thing! Hypnopoetic. Congratulations *bobser*. ☺

KELLEY T WOODS (Hypnotherapist)

I find Bob Burn's *Swan* to be totally delightful and have applied it for a wide spectrum of clients, from ages 6 to 87! I consider myself a teacher and encourage clients to use the things they learn to continue to improve, even when they are no longer with me, so it's always a joy when clients return and comment on how their Swan helped them in their everyday experience. This amazing video clearly demonstrates several valuable lessons, to wit, 1) no expectancy of outcome doesn't mean we don't learn something 2) the need to be patient and allow for time to respond 3) the importance to ask the SC to play (how many people, practitioners and clients, spend time worrying about what they are afraid might happen, instead of asking for what they want to happen?!) 4) how we can employ utilization for the client's benefit 5) how wonderful it is to ratify experience by transitioning into deeper experiences.

MATIC MATO SUMRADA (Slovenia)

Holy s**t Bob, I just watched The Swan again and tried to test if my subconscious will react just by listening to you...and it did...and I freaked out! That is amazing! I didn't get the first twitch, but the turn was huge, almost 160° turn. And my arm still feels funny, like I don't have control over it. The DVD is great and worth every penny.

SHANA ROOMERS (therapist, Belgium)

Hi Everybody, Yesterday I had someone that was completely emotionally entangled. trust problems, communication problems, and a very low self-esteem. She really wanted to know where the problem came from. I used The Swan and had the characters for Yes / No / I don't know. In the analysis of what the problems are, I asked the subconscious to give a sign to the conscious mind, but it couldn't do this. I asked whether this was possible in hypnosis, and then it told me that it was possible! So, I proceeded with hypnosis and then return immediately to resume with the Swan into the hypnosis where the subconscious could make immediate contact with the conscious mind! I then proceeded with regression, using the Swan. And *wauwww* that was super!! Every time I asked to bring her to a new place in time, I asked the subconscious to turn the wrist inside and back outside so I could see that she had arrived on the spot. Meanwhile, I was able to ask questions of both consciousness *(with direct voice!!!),* what they saw and felt, etc. .. as talk to the subconscious (whether this was really the first place, or if there are other related things to the problem, etc) It was very nice to do, you could talk with the two! Super to do and great result. Everything was reset with tears of happiness. Afterwards I asked if the subconscious could give her a super strong feeling and give her a very big smile on her face. And it did! Then I also asked the subconscious to let her get up in the morning every day with that big smile and that also was no problem!! All if this... All in one session!!! Swan + regression = match made in heaven!

Thank you, Bob Burns.

DAVID OST An amazing experience thanks to The Swan I did it and that hand couldn't move any further as I spotted my client closing his eyes and heard the voice of a tiny little boy trying to talk to me. I instructed his subconscious to take over his voice and his body if he wanted to talk to me in order to help him overcome a trauma of his childhood..... It did!!! He began saying that he was afraid of men and so on. This boy was sexually abused by another man. I made it clear that it all belonged to the past and instructed him to 'let go' all the pain etc. with every breath he would take. I also taught him to feel good and happy every time he'd open a door. At a certain moment I let the little boy go 'hide' himself in the client. My client woke up and knew nothing about what had happened! When I told him some private things the little boy had told me (and the client hadn't told me anything before) he was puzzled. This man was amazed and felt really well for the first time in his life (he's 39!). Afterwards he told me he was sceptic, but that he was very satisfied he came to me. It was again a beautiful experience I wanted to share with you all. Just to let you know these things can really happen. Thank you so much Bob Burns.

STEVE SHELDON

Yep I had the thought of *do* The Swan then bang em in. Well what a surprise I got. My client didn't just bang in or relax in. She was fine with The Swan but not hypnosis. So, I did everything through The Swan. I do want to say thanks Bob Burns, you gave me things to change and to think about. Also, I am a swanner now!! Lol

CLAUDIA KNICHEL

Had a fantastic session! The Swan started to talk to me whilst I just thought & felt about it. We had two lovely Swans and two parts and the Swans did all kind of movement, even dancing, flipping, rolling around each other, etc. - and all without me telling them, simply playing their own game. A huge change already in Session 1 with the client being absolutely fascinated and truly happy afterwards.

IRWIN LEPMA

Boy what a difference! My clients and I as a hypnotist, hypnosis experience that is sooo intense, so powerful. The Swan as an introduction to the whole process, as the use of anabolic steroids in hypnosis. The feedback I get from my clients is that the session touched them to the bone, emotional and surprised at their own subconscious. I cannot other than to say a big Thank you, to you, Bob Burns, for this amazing tool '

HELEN LEURINK

Yesterday session done with only The Swan, no hypnosis thereafter. Went really great. Fantastic movements. Lady had written down in advance what they would like changed & wanted to have. Worked really fine. Super awesome.!!!!!

JOLANDA HUNTER

This afternoon made a hypnosis session, customer with vertigo. Started with the Swan and got super response, beautiful hand turned to face to clear yes and no finger. In my view the problem was gone. During hypnosis again used the Swan and received confirmation that the problem is solved. I mean... how great is that!

RINKE JACOBS

Beautiful Swan today when trying to remember memories. The beauty of it all, I think that connecting that reaction that one perceives can be reassigned to the fact that the suggestions at that time had already come into effect. Beautiful!

MARIELLE VANHOEF

The first Swan is a fact, I'm a fan! It seems like hocus-pocus ... amazing. Feeling excited!!!

HELEEN BORNEMAN

Wow, wow, wow!! Today, a really great experience with the Swan! Never before had such a violent *Swan* reaction. My client was very hard to get the last time. Hypnosis was very much in control. Today I thought I'm SWANNING. Well good thing! She was not there and I got me a spasm on all sides. The client was really scared of the reaction of her hand and compared it with horror even, she thought it was so scary. Her hand shook with a spasm in fingers and yes in no fingers also from a spasm. She also said she even felt the cramp inside her lap and she was sometimes concerned with the question, and they all felt the fingers constrict. For her and for me a great experience with all the consequences for the section where I sit with this client. Thank you for this fantastic method!

LIZA HOEK

Wow, what an addition to the hypnosis session with The Swan! Today I had two clients. The latter was a young man with many fears and hypochondriac symptoms. He does not trust his body. After the session, he was out of the blue!

AMANDA BOUMAN

The Swan... Pure pleasure. Lol. Talk to the hand the face Is not listening. I tell my client, Do you feel like something fun to do? To experience something beautiful and something a little crazy .... Of course they do. It is amazing!!!

Paul Mischel

Client, Female, late 50's from Australia. Presenting issue, Peripheral neuropathy, that persisted 24 hours a day without abatement. Diagnosed by her General Practitioner as stemming from Lyme disease.

Case history: She had been bitten by a tick in Central Queensland approximately 5 years prior and had been experiencing symptoms of a Lyme like disease since that initial bite. The Australian Health Department doesn't recognise the presence of Lyme disease in Australia, as it has not been detected in native Australian ticks, although people in Australia are experiencing Lyme like symptoms. Her bloodwork had been sent off to Germany by her GP to ascertain the presence of Borrelia burgdorferi, a bacterium linked with Lyme disease. The German lab had returned a positive result for the presence of the bacteria. Lyme disease is a controversial area of medicine in Australia and this documentary on Australian Lyme Disease sufferers may provide you with additional context on how challenging it is for this type of client to get treatment and support, let alone a resolution. The Australian Medical Association refuses to acknowledge this is an issue and this is a report outlining its stance on the matter – Treatment: After taking a thorough case history, I proceeded to initiate the Swan protocol. I received a very animated response from her Swan. She showed positive signs for the twitch, turn, wave, return and Yes / No responses. I simply asked her Swan if the peripheral neuropathy served any important purpose for her? Her Swan responded with a "No". I then asked it if it would be OK, if the peripheral neuropathy was removed from her experience? Her Swan responded with a "Yes". I then requested that it please remove the peripheral neuropathy, and signal Yes when it was done. From initial questioning of her Swan to resolution, it was about 20-30 seconds maximum. When her yes finger twitched, she looked around the clinic room in bewilderment. I asked her what she was looking for, to which she responded, *"It just vanished, where did it go?"* I asked her, *"What vanished?"* And she responded, *"The pain, it just disappeared"*. Despite her adherence to the idea that the peripheral neuropathy was caused by Lyme disease, she walked out of the clinic pain free for the first time in 5 years. We had a follow up session a month later at her request. She had experienced a stressful life experience and the peripheral neuropathy had returned. I ran the same process from the previous session and asked her Swan to find other more useful ways of managing distress and within 10 seconds the peripheral neuropathy had gone! To my knowledge she has been pain free ever since the session with no return of the peripheral neuropathy.

David Wynn (Spain)

I use the Swan almost every single day. At first, I didn't get what could be regarded as consistent results. Now it just seems to work virtually every time! I guess it's because I truly believe in what I'm doing and I think maybe the hidden antenna of my clients picks that up? I don't know but it is without doubt a beautiful method of working with clients as well as being a great convincer. I do a lot of quit smoking work, (not at your prices Bob 😊) but I demonstrate the Swan with every single one of them before I do traditional hypnosis. I use it as part of my pretalk stating that since entering the room I have been talking directly to the subconscious and every time they have nodded or said yes you have confirmed your true desire for change. I then say I'm so convinced of this that I think I could communicate directly with their deeper mind without any hypnosis whatsoever!!! They look at me strangely and it then begins. The work is done before the trance is started. As I'm finishing the Swan and before hypnosis, I even apologise to the *unconscious* stating I may be repeating some things in Hypnosis and please forgive me but it's for the client's benefit. The client listens on and is completely confident by this time that they will never smoke (or whatever) again. A month ago, I had a lady visit me with severe anxiety. To such a point every morning her stomach was knotted, it felt like being sick and felt terrible. I did my pretalk and finished with the Swan. She has written to me several times, stating that her anxiety had completely gone, huge changes taking place in her life and after her last visit the following day she cried for four hours solid without knowing why! I still haven't done any therapeutic work with traditional hypnosis. I cannot underestimate the amazing self-curing power people can obtain with The Swan. The lady had been suffering for over 5 years and being extremely wealthy had seen the best psychologists and doctors in the country and *many* of them. It took The Swan and 70 euros to sort it!!! 😊 Every day I feel blessed thankful and I must admit a touch proud to use this process and help so many people. No bullshit mate, it's fucking amazing. [that was not a typo. 😊] It is my intention that everyone gets to hear and use The Swan. At least in Spain and anywhere else where Spanish is spoken.

ALEX VRETTOS

Often when learning a new technique, I have found it necessary to fail with it before achieving a perfect result... but in the case of The Swan I hit the ground running! A client who we can call Roger got in touch with me as he was learning to drive quite late in his life but experiencing panic attacks behind the wheel of a car. He did not know why but did mention he had a sledging accident when he was 15 and wondered if it had anything to do with that. Once we were fully acquainted, I lifted his hand into position feeling that familiar feeling of nervous excitement. I invited the part to come and talk to me using his hand and almost immediately his hand turned towards him in a way that made me think of a naked Emu on Rod Hull's lap! Roger screamed and nearly fell off his chair and I nearly joined him as laughter erupted from deep inside me! Bob's right. It IS great to have fun in the therapy room. When we had regained our composure Roger's hand was swinging between us both as if waiting for one of us to speak and so I took charge. We established yes and no signals and a very definite willingness to speak to me using his voice. The word Hello emanated very quickly from his mouth in a much deeper and raspier voice than Roger's. "Do you have a name or title you wish to be known by?" I asked. "Shadow," the part said. At this point, if we had not been at my own house I think I would have run away and never come back, but I stuck with it. "Shadow?" I said. "That's an interesting name. Why Shadow?" "Because I am always lurking." Still resisting a powerful urge to leave, I asked, "Great. Do you have a particular role in Roger's life?" "Yes. I am the caretaker." I had no idea where this was going but this is the beauty of The Swan. I find that so long as you remain clever and relevant with your questions you end up exactly where you need to be. "And what does being the caretaker involve?" I asked. "Well I'm always clearing up after him aren't I." Now this was starting to make some sense. It turned out the panic attacks were Shadow's doing and it did have something to do with the sledging accident, but we never mentioned driving again. Shadow told me it wanted to retire but did not know how and so agreed to let me help. It was not ready to go yet and needed a couple of weeks to 'tie up its affairs'. I ended the session and Roger came back to the conversation delighted with the experience. I told him that we would hopefully complete things in a second session in two weeks' time. Two weeks later I reconnected with Shadow who said he was ready but was a bit fidgety and nervous about going. It said it had made all its necessary arrangements and so I started to talk it through finding the light and going into the light. Shadow got more and more fidgety though and said it could not find the light as it lived in the shadows. I therefore asked to speak to another part of Roger's mind who could help us. His higher self came through, a very chatty and officious part, who said, "Yes Shadow needs to go, he really needs to go, he is so old, he is just holding us all back."

184

I explained our predicament stopping Shadow from leaving and the higher self agreed to 'knock a hole in the ceiling' so the light can get through. He did this and told me when it was done. I spoke to Shadow again who was completely chilled now and told me it had found the light and it was beautiful. I told him to go into the light and take all its worries with it as the light will dissolve them. As I spoke, Roger's head slumped further and further forwards and so I gave him suggestions that the further into the light Shadow went, the closer back to the room Roger could drift. Roger's head lifted, his eyes opened. "That was amazing!" he said, and the panic attacks stopped!

And finally, from someone who simply wrote: "As I said when we met Bob, I have my thing and you have yours. The difference being I have made a fortune with my thing whilst yours, properly used, might save the world. But both of our gifts will hopefully open up the minds of humanity. Good luck on your travels 'Swan Man'. Much love,
"Uri" x

Chapter 13

Swan cheat sheet

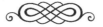

SWAN INCIDENTALS (the *cheat sheet* given out during workshops)

Here is the exact wording Bob Burns uses in every single Swan Session, and for good reasons.
(However, do remember The Goldilocks Principle, so you will not be phased by any of the following ☺).

The Swan Protocol should always be prefixed by and include 6 incidentals:
1) a gathering of (small amount) information
2) a statement of wonder
3) a statement of fact (followed by a question of confirmation)
4) enquiry re: their manual and which is their dominant hand
5) 3 instructions
6) 3 suggestions
7) Swan Contact

1]
The Gathering of Information
(although this is also the start of The Consultation it is added here because often you will ONLY be doing… The Swan)
This is about asking why they are here **today** (today being the operative word) as there might have been a recent happening which you need to know about in order to ascertain their actual problem (we find that, in reality, nobody ever comes to a hypnotherapist with a CONSCIOUS problem!)

2]
The Statement of Wonder
… is made AFTER gathering a small but sufficient amount of information, which prompts the therapist to say:
"Well, the good news is that you don't actually have a problem!
That is... not a CONSCIOUS problem. Rather yours is a SUBconscious problem, which tells me that it's all INSIDE of you, yet totally OUTSIDE of your control.... would that be about right?"
(and watch how they always say yes).
Remember, that if THEY say it, only THEN does it become true!).
It's funny but all over the world, in workshops, the students continually ask:
"What happens if they DON'T confirm that: 'YES, this IS the case?' That they don't have a conscious problem, but rather it is: 'a SUBconscious problem, all inside them yet totally outside their control'.
... and the annoying answer [LOL] I promise you, is that it never EVER happens!!!
And even if it DID happen then that would mean that the therapist has erred in either: hesitation, modulation, emphasis or inflection
(in their presentation of the question).

3]

A Statement of Fact (followed by confirmation)
"So if you don't have a conscious problem but rather a subconscious problem then that means I'm probably wasting my time talking to YOU. But rather I'd be far better talking to that part within your SUBconscious which understands just what the problem is. Maybe when, why and how it was caused and how it can be helped or even fixed! Does THAT make sense, yeah?"
(again look for that confirmation).

4]
Enquiry re: Manual and Dominant Hand
A) "Did you bring you manual with you? No? Pity. Wouldn't it be great if you simply walked in the door, told me what's bothering you and then handed me your manual in order that I could look it up in order to follow the instructions on how to fix you.
So if you don't have a manual (smile) that means I have to fidget (the word *ficher* is used in Scotland) a little with you, in order to find out just how you work, yeah?

B) "Tell me, are you right or left handed ? Great, so put your left hand like this (shape of The Swan)"
And of course whatever they answer the therapist (assuming the therapist uses their own right hand, chooses the client's LEFT hand) solely for the purpose of symmetry).

5]
3 Instructions
"So three things:
I don't want you to fight me.
But I don't want you to help me either.
Rather you simply allow me to work, okay?"
and then…
"So, your job… is to do nothing! So what's YOUR job?"
That last question (as important as it IS) I feel can *only* be for the therapist who is comfortable within their own 'bedside manner'. It should be said with a smile and/or a shrug, and obviously NOT in a condescending way. ☺

6]
3 Suggestions
"One of three things is now about to happen. The first is, as crazy as this sounds, your hand will move, all on its own.
The second thing is that your hand won't move, but you'll feel it trying to move.
And of course the third thing could be that not only will it not move but you won't feel anything either.

And all of that is okay, as it simply tells me a little more of how you work, I simply get feedback. Is that okay?"

7]
SWAN CONTACT!
(assumed name of client is Sue)
"Great! So remember Sue, I'm now going to totally ignore you, so excuse my bad manners. I'm simply going to talk to that part inside you, and see what happens… (when they acknowledge… turn and face the hand)
Understand that unlike most hypnotic protocols rather than coerce, cajole or motivate, with The Swan there doesn't have to be A Pitch. Indeed the therapist can even appear quite pessimistic!

Bob Burns has a favourite line with all clients and indeed students:
"I'm very pessimistic in the therapy room by the way.
I've had to actually train myself to be that way, since I discovered over many years that being optimistic brought me many disappointments, whilst being pessimistic got me no disappointments, yet many wonderful surprises.
But I'm not a negative pessimist. I am indeed a very positive pessimist!"
(said with a smile. *Always* with a smile).

This does 2 things. First it immediately lessens the impact of potential failure (acting as an *out* for worst case scenario) in order that although there might *be* a failure… is not actually *recognized* as failure.
It also acts as a form of intended confusion like that of a witchdoctoring technique, inasmuch that the client will often smile in disbelief that such a statement could even be made by a therapist in a therapy room. But I honestly believe that this has the power to build counter expectancy ("would he really say that unless he *knew* something?").
Remember, we are NOT seeking any form of social compliance. On the contrary we MUST destroy it if at all possible. It's not a somnambulistic circus. We want to KNOW if we are *winning*, and not just *looking good*?

"So hi (said to The Swan), I'm not talking to Sue anymore, I'm talking to you. I want you to know that I see you, I believe in you, and I want to talk to you!
Now you can either do this or you can't, or you want to do it or you don't. But let's find out…shall we?
I want you please to simply tweak one of Sue's fingers… it might be a forefinger that wants to lift or curl, or maybe even the small finger… or a thumb… that's right"

IF the finger moves we say 'to Sue':
"You're not doing that just to please me are you (seeking confirmation that no social compliance is taking place)?"
If no movement takes place we say (to Sue):
"Tell me can you feel anything happening within any of the fingers?"
Regardless of the answer we then say:
"You might find this interesting……"
(this again is intentionally an OPEN statement)
… before turning back to The Swan and saying:
"So now… I want you to go into Sue's entire hand, and arm, and simply turn it like this (showing with your mirroring arm) *around towards her face. Do that for me now please…. Thankyou!"*
(So if the fingers do not move, we *totally ignore that* and carry on. Very often although the fingers fail to move the hand will! And don't forget to be using a language that includes PLEASE and THANKYOU)

After the turn:
"That's lovely, thankyou. And now can I ask, if you were to say 'HELLO' to Sue, how exactly would you DO that? I mean would you be able to wave the whole hand? Or would it simply be a finger that moves? Can you show me how please?"
This of course will be seen by many as totally ridiculous, which of course makes any movement totally *miraculous*.
If no movement ask the client:
"And tell me Sue, could you feeeeeeeel something going on there?"
Now address The Swan:
"Thankyou, and now I'd very much like you to take Sue's hand and that whole arm and turn everything all the way back to face me please. SO you're now having to find and use different

190

nerves, fibres and muscles."
If it's taking some time then prompt with:
"… and you may have to work this out yes? I realize you've never been asked to do this before… so do take your time… that's right…" etc
By this time the therapist should be extreeeeeeeemely comfortable with both the client and 'the caller/part' however the last part of this initial teaching of The Swan is to go for what some people might wish to term: an ideo-motor response (IMR).

The therapist then continues with the final three questions before conversation can be initiated:
1) *"So if I asked you a question and the answer was YES can you show me how you would say yes to me? Would it be a nodding hand or the lifting of a particular finger…?"*
2) *"Thankyou and how might you say NO to me?"*
3) *"And if you wished to convey that you either didn't KNOW or were UNSURE how would you convey that to me?"*
Then you may feel free to begin questions…

This concludes the *cheat sheet* for The (basic) Swan Protocol.

However…. Why not try for…. Direct Voice!
Still to The Swan…
"I was just wondering, if you can move a finger, a hand or a whole arm… can you do more… (rhetorical)… would you be happy to try more?
For example, and I'm not asking you to DO it, I just want to know if you could, and if you'd like to.
If it were possible for you to (you look as if you are in deep thought)*…*
…SPEAK… to me… do you think you could…..?

Be comfortable in the silence. This will often be one of the biggest moments of their lives…

Would you like to try…..?
Would you like to try now…?

(big smile and perhaps a gentle touch of an arm, as you get client agreement)
"Are you okay with this Sue?"

Back to The Swan…
"So, when you're ready, in your own time. Just allow yourself to take control of Sue's cardiovascular system, her heart, her lungs, her mouth. her tongue. And when YOU are ready, just take a nice deep breath and simply say the word… Hello!"

…..and when this happens for the first time, you, as a therapist… will simply explode! 😊

Close

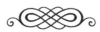

And so, I do hope you've learned something new from this wee book, or maybe reminded you of something you forgot along the way? Or that I've possibly sent you off on a new line of thought. Hopefully we'll meet again in my next book where I'll be sharing some new and fascinating ideas and some stories that I've never got round to sharing before. Hopefully several that will make you smile. Remember, they simply can't stop us laughing!!! 😊

Until then,

Yours aye,

Bob Burns

Web Links

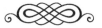

Page 81. business Card   **https://youtu.be/CvUD41syEEs**

Page 117. Chevreul's Pendulum   **https://youtu.be/fLek_wIucJU**

Page 126. First 3 response tests   **https://youtu.be/Htdof83iOOU**

Page 127. successful hand stick   **https://youtu.be/ag-VpKu7C-Q**

Page 127. unsuccessful hand stick   **https://youtu.be/3-ouURFheTE**

Page 131. Induction   **https://youtu.be/SzC5O8cS6-k**

Page 135. Cascade   **https://youtu.be/t9d9rtyGSRw**

Page 136. Relaxation   **https://youtu.be/KtwVoFHL_9g**

Page 153. Stop It!   **https://youtu.be/Ow0lr63y4Mw**

Page. 163 The Battleship   **https://youtu.be/zns4cqkirMQ**

Printed in Great Britain
by Amazon

11757009R00112